Textbook of Community Ophthalmology

This book presents a comprehensive treatise on ~~~~~~~~~~~~~ ~lmology principles and practices for countries with developing and emerging economies. It is replete with chapters on basic epidemiology, health economics, and basic statistics and lays the foundation of the global eye healthcare programmes with skills for community-based epidemiological projects in eye care. With extensive experience in conducting various epidemiological surveys funded by the Ministry of Health, WHO, Indian Council of Medical Research, etc., the editors provide practical knowledge to ophthalmologists, public health specialists, physician-scientists, researchers, eye care programme managers, optometrists, and academicians involved in community ophthalmology operational studies.

Key Features:

- Presents a single platform for knowing everything about community ophthalmology, from statistics and epidemiology to financing, in an easy and succinct manner.
- Serves as a robust resource and an advanced teaching tool for medical professionals.
- Includes well-illustrated, succinct chapters for better understanding of various aspects of public health in eye care.
- Provides tips and tricks for dealing with both expected and unexpected situations while conducting epidemiological research and data collection in the field.

Textbook of Community Ophthalmology

Edited by

Praveen Vashist

MD, MSc. CEH (LSHTM, London)
Professor and Head of Community Ophthalmology
Dr R. P. Centre for Ophthalmic Sciences,
All India Institute of Medical Sciences, New Delhi, India

Noopur Gupta

MS, DNB, MNAMS, PhD
Additional Professor of Ophthalmology,
Dr R. P. Centre for Ophthalmic Sciences,
All India Institute of Medical Sciences, New Delhi, India

Suraj Singh Senjam

MBBS, MD (PGI, Chand), MSc. PHEC (LSHTM, London)
Professor of Community Ophthalmology
Dr R. P. Centre for Ophthalmic Sciences,
All India Institute of Medical Sciences, New Delhi, India

Vivek Gupta

MBBS, MD, MSc. PHEC (LSHTM, London)
Additional Professor, Community Ophthalmology
Dr R. P. Centre for Ophthalmic Sciences,
All India Institute of Medical Sciences, New Delhi, India

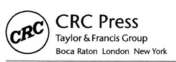

CRC Press is an imprint of the
Taylor & Francis Group, an **informa** business

Designed cover image: Shutterstock

First edition published 2024
by CRC Press
6000 Broken Sound Parkway NW, Suite 300, Boca Raton, FL 33487–2742

and by CRC Press
4 Park Square, Milton Park, Abingdon, Oxon, OX14 4RN

CRC Press is an imprint of Taylor & Francis Group, LLC

© 2024 selection and editorial matter, Praveen Vashist, Noopur Gupta, Suraj Singh Senjam and Vivek Gupta; individual chapters, the contributors

ISBN: 9781032271590 (hbk)
ISBN: 9781032271583 (pbk)
ISBN: 9781003291626 (ebk)

DOI: 10.1201/9781003291626

Typeset in Minion
by Apex CoVantage, LLC

Contents

Foreword

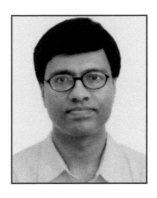

 अखिल भारतीय आयुर्विज्ञान संस्थान **All India Institute of Medical Sciences**
अंसारी नगर, नई दिल्ली-110029, भारत Ansari Nagar, New Delhi-110029, India

It is with immense pleasure that I am writing the Foreword for this much-needed and much-awaited excellent textbook for community ophthalmology for not just ophthalmology residents and fellows but also for community medicine residents as a reference guide. Community ophthalmology is mainly aimed at people-centric preventive care rather than person-centric curative care and aimed at the community at large. The main aim of this book is to guide the readers on various aspects of community ophthalmology right from its inception to its recent progress in preventing avoidable blindness and visual impairment. The leaps and bounds in this area are explicitly shown by a reduction of avoidable blindness in India and have been possible with implementation of the many aspects of community ophthalmology and its preventive measures for improving ocular health in the community at large.

This book has been drafted in 13 well-written chapters by some of the stalwarts in the field. Dr Praveen Vashist and his team have worked hard to write, assemble, and edit the contributions of a much-renowned and distinguished group of experts to come out with this excellent and unique text. They have covered a wide array of topics ranging from the basics of epidemiology right to the details of health economics and teleophthalmology, which was the need of the hour during the COVID-19 pandemic.

I extend my hearty congratulations to all the authors for their contributions, and the editors for their commendable work in systematically compiling and editing the text, ensuring completeness, comprehensiveness, and quality of the work. Finally, I would like to extend my best wishes to them for all the success in their efforts and recommend this excellent textbook to all those interested in the field of public health for eye care, especially community ophthalmology. I have no doubt that the *Textbook of Community Ophthalmology* will be a very valuable addition to all the libraries in medical institutions as well as the governing bodies related to public health.

M. Srinivas, MCh
Director
AIIMS, New Delhi

Preface

The first edition of *Textbook of Community Ophthalmology* is dedicated to all the community experts, clinicians, and scientists who have contributed to the education in our field of medical students, residents, and fellows, and especially to all the community ophthalmologists who have participated in continuing medical education. Community ophthalmology is an upcoming field which aims at prevention of disease at community level.

The *Textbook of Community Ophthalmology* is intended to provide a concise and comprehensive resource for individuals with an interest in the field of community ophthalmology. Community ophthalmology deals with the delivery of eye care with the involvement of preventive, curative, promotive, and rehabilitation activities, making it a holistic approach towards eye care with clinical ophthalmology at its core. Comprehensive eye care service involves approaches in preventing eye diseases and must begin where people live and work. The need to be constantly in touch with the population and to consistently update about their eye care status is a reflection of the rapid pace of progress in our efforts to reduce avoidable blindness not just in one individual but in the entire community at large. Despite its importance in a developing country like India, community ophthalmology departments are rare even in the best of tertiary care hospitals. Dr Rajendra Prasad Centre for Ophthalmic Sciences, AIIMS, New Delhi, has provided us with the platform to move ahead with important national and regional surveys and interventions targeting avoidable blindness, visual impairment, low vision and rehabilitation, health education, and in general, promoting eye health in the community. It has been this platform that inspired the idea of this book.

The editorial team for this book has been immensely thorough in the chapters to help clarify the respective topics at hand. The edition has also benefitted from a talented group of contributing authors from across the country. We are certainly grateful to them for sharing their expertise and wisdom in the pages of this text. It should be noted that our authors have extensive and outstanding expertise to be a part of this book and worked under extraordinary circumstances, such as the global coronavirus pandemic. Our book was developed in the midst of the greatest healthcare challenge the world has faced in over a century. The COVID-19 pandemic nearly brought our community work to a halt. Thus, we dedicate our book not only to the frontline healthcare workers who worked tirelessly to save each precious life but also to the tremendous work of scientists all around the world who put forth vaccines which helped save countless lives. We dedicate ourselves and our work for the betterment of our society and hope to continue working for the benefit of the community.

Praveen Vashist, MD
Noopur Gupta, MS, PhD
Suraj Singh Senjam, MD
Vivek Gupta, MD

About the Editors

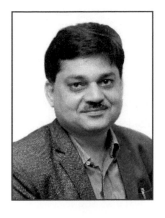

Dr Praveen Vashist is the head of community ophthalmology, Dr Rajendra Prasad Centre for Ophthalmic Sciences, All India Institute of Medical Sciences, New Delhi. He is a public health expert and has post-graduate degree in community medicine from LHMC, New Delhi, and has completed his master's degree in community eye health from London School of Hygiene and Tropical Medicine (LSHTM), London. He has been instrumental in developing community outreach programs along with strengthening epidemiological research and training in the field of community eye care. He has contributed immensely towards the development of health policies as a key resource person for technical support for National Programme for Control of Blindness in India. He is the vice president and a key resource person for Vision 2020: The Right to Sight, India.

As a principal investigator, he has led all major surveys over the last decade under NPCB&VI, which includes the National Blindness and Visual Impairment Surveys, National Diabetic Retinopathy Surveys, National Trachoma Prevalence and Rapid Assessment Surveys, National Human Resource and Infrastructure Survey, and the development of India Vision Atlas. Currently, he is leading the NPCB&VI National Trachomatous Trichiasis surveys conducted in 200 previously trachoma-endemic districts in the country. His ardent interest in the field of research and community eye care is clearly evident in his more than 100 publications in international and national journals.

He serves as an international expert to the WHO SAERO and WHO Geneva and coordinates WHO collaborating centre activities in R. P. Centre. He was a member of the dossier review committee for validation of trachoma elimination in Nepal and Myanmar. He was awarded the 2023 Achievement Award in the 38th Asia-Pacific Academy of Ophthalmology. He was also honoured with the AIIMS Excellence Research Award in 2014 and 2017, the ACOIN Gold Medal, the G. Venkataswamy Memorial Award, and the Best Community Ophthalmology Paper in AIOS.

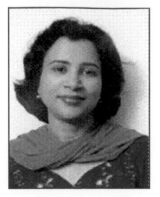

Dr Noopur Gupta, MS (Gold Medal, Lady Hardinge Medical College, New Delhi, India), DNB, MNAMS, PhD (Community Ophthalmology, AIIMS), is an eminent member of the cornea, cataract, and refractive surgery services at Dr Rajendra Prasad Centre for Ophthalmic Sciences, All India Institute of Medical Sciences, New Delhi, India. With nearly 20 years of teaching and research experience, she has actively participated as a chairperson, instructor, judge, and faculty at various regional, national, and international conferences. She has received numerous awards at national and international platforms for robust public health research, including the Excellence in Ophthalmic Research (All India Ophthalmology Conference) and AIIMS Excellence Awards. She received the ORBIS International Medal at Barcelona, Spain, for best paper contributing to prevention of blindness in the developing world for her work on keratomalacia. Her contributions in the field of cornea, dry eye disease, and community ophthalmology have been lauded both nationally and globally.

With more than 200 publications to her credit, she is a reviewer and editor of many national and international journals and has contributed immensely to national health policies and advocacy. She has been the key ophthalmologist and trainer for national-level blindness and trachoma surveys supported by the Ministry of Health and Family Welfare, Government of India. She serves as an international expert to the World Health Organization, Geneva, and has actively contributed to developing recommendations for global elimination of neglected tropical diseases.

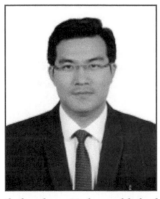

Dr Suraj Singh Senjam is a professor currently working in the community ophthalmology section at Dr R. P. Centre for Ophthalmic Sciences, All India Institute of Medical Sciences, New Delhi. He earned his post-graduate degree in community medicine from PGIMER, Chandigarh, and completed his master's degree in public health for eye care from the London School of Hygiene and Tropical Medicine (LSHTM), London. He was one of the awardees of ASIA-ARVO 2013 New Delhi for his poster presentation and received the best free paper presentation in AIOC 2019 for social ophthalmology. He has published more than 80 research papers in national and international peer-reviewed indexed journals. He has established the Vision Rehabilitation and Training Centre in community ophthalmology and led a winning low-vision rehabilitation programme in South-East Asia with support from the WHO South-East Asia regional office. He has led the Rapid Assistive Technology Assessment (rATA) study in India, supported by the WHO Geneva. He also received the best government assistive initiative in the government sector organized by IIT Madras. He is one of the key investigators for the National Blindness Survey in 30 districts supported by the Ministry of Health, Government of India.

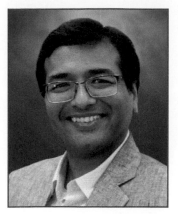

Dr Vivek Gupta is a graduate of the University College of Medical Sciences, Delhi, and an MD (Community Medicine) from AIIMS, New Delhi, in 2005. He has over 15 years of experience as a public health specialist. Since 2015, he has been engaged as a faculty of community ophthalmology at Dr Rajendra Prasad Centre for Ophthalmic Sciences. He has 85+ PubMed indexed publications, with 2,600+ citations, h-index of 23, and i10-index of 48. He is a recipient of AIOS ET Selvam Award 2017, Commonwealth Scholarship 2021, LSHTM Gordon Jhonson Award 2022, LSHTM Hooper Award 2022 and is a fellow of Dr Ramachandra N Moorthy Foundation for Mental Health and Neurological Sciences. He is a co-investigator of the National Blindness and Visual Impairment Survey, National Diabetic Retinopathy Survey, National Trachoma Survey, National Eye Care HR and Infrastructure Survey, and Cause of Death Ascertainment through Verbal Autopsies under SRS for the Registrar General of India. Prior work has included contributions to non-communicable diseases, respiratory diseases, National Mental Health Survey, and public health interventions for tuberculosis. He is interested in blindness survey methodologies, myopia epidemiology, trachoma, health information systems, and prevention and leveraging technology for improving public health.

Contributors

Kowsalya Akkayasamy
Neuro-ophthalmologist in Aravind Eye
Care System, Madurai
Chinthamani Madurai, Tamil Nadu, India

Amit Bhardwaj MSW
Medical Social Service Officer
All India Institute of Medical Sciences,
New Delhi, India

Monica Chaudhary
MCVI and Founder Learn Beyond Vision
1106, Sector 15-Part 2, Gurgram,
Haryana-122001, India

Mohammed Gowth Amanullah
Lions Aravind Institute of Community
Ophthalmology
Aravind Eye Care System, Madurai,
India

**Sumit Grover DO, DNB (Ophthal.),
FICO (UK) MBA (Hospital
Management) MSc. PHEC, LSHTM
(Univ. of London)**
Assistant Professor of Ophthalmology
AIIMS, New Delhi (NCI Jhajjar
Campus), India

**Sumit Malhotra MD (Community
Medicine, AIIMS), DNB (Social and
Preventive Medicine)**
Associate Professor
Centre for Community Medicine
All India Institute of Medical Sciences
(AIIMS), New Delhi, India

Souvik Manna MBBS, MD, MIPHA
Member, International Epidemiological
Association
PhD Scholar, AIIMS, New Delhi,
India

Sunny Mannava MPH
Research Scholar (PhD, Public Health)
School of Medical Sciences
University of Hyderabad
Hyderabad, India

G. V. S. Murthy, MSc, MD, MBBS
Director
Indian Institute of Public Health–
Hyderabad
Amar Co-op Society
Kavuri Hills, Madhapur
Hyderabad, India

Phanindra Babu Nukella
PhD, Chief Executive Officer
Vision 2020: The Right to Sight,
India

**Nawazish Shaikh MD
(Ophthalmology), DNB**
Research Officer (Medical)
Community Ophthalmology
All India Institute of Medical Sciences,
New Delhi, India

B. R. Shamanna
Professor, School of Medical Sciences
University of Hyderabad
Gachibowli, Hyderabad, India

Meera Sharma MSW
Research Officer (Non-Medical)
Community Ophthalmology
All India Institute of Medical Sciences,
New Delhi, India

Pallavi Shukla MD (Community Medicine), PhD
Preventive Oncology, IRCH
All India Institute of Medical Sciences,
New Delhi, India

Meenakshi Wadhwani MS, PGDHM (NIHFW), PhD
Assistant Professor and In-Charge
Paediatric Ophthalmology
Chacha Nehru Bal Chikitsalya,
New Delhi, India

Abbreviations

ASHA	Accredited Social Health Activist
ADL	Activities of Daily Living
ARMD	Age-Related Macular Degeneration
ANTI-VEGF	Anti-Vascular Endothelial Growth Factor
ADIP	Assistance to Disabled Persons for Purchase/Fitting of Aids and Appliances
AR	Attributable Risk
ANM	Auxiliary Nurse Midwife
ACER	Average Cost-Effectiveness Ratio
AB-HWC	Ayushman Bharat Health and Wellness Centre
BRAC	Bangladesh Rehabilitation Assistance Committee
BCC	Behavioural Change Communication
BCR	Benefit–Cost Ratio
BCVA	Best Corrected Visual Acuity
BEMP	Biomedical Equipment Maintenance Programme
BMI	Body Mass Index
CBBF	Cataract Blindness Backlog Free
CSR	Cataract Surgical Rate
CSS	Centrally Sponsored Schemes
COE	Centres of Excellence
CLS	Cluster Sampling
CBR	Community-Based Rehabilitation
CHC	Community Health Centre
CHO	Community Health Officer
CNAA	Community Needs Assessment Approach
CHEERS 2022	Consolidated Health Economic Evaluation Reporting Standards 2022
CME	Continuing Medical Education
CO	Corneal Opacity
C	Cortex
CBA	Cost–Benefit Analysis
CEA	Cost-Effectiveness Ratio
CUA	Cost–Utility Analysis
CIR	Crude Incidence Rate

DDG	Deputy Director General
DR	Diabetic Retinopathy
DALY	Disability-Adjusted Life Years
DPO	Disabled Persons Organization
DBCS	District Blindness Control Societies
DHS	District Health Societies
DH	District Hospital
DPC	District Planning Committee
EMGT	Early Manifest Glaucoma Trial
EVI	Early Visual Impairment
ECSC	Effective Cataract Surgery Coverage
EREC	Effective Refractive Error Coverage
EDC	Electronic Data Collection
EMR	Electronic Medical Records
EM	Expectation Maximization
FRU	First Referral Units
FGD	Focused Group Discussions
FDT	Frequency Doubling Technology (Perimetry)
FLV	Functional Low Vision
GEE	Generalized Estimating Equations
GAP	Global Action Plan
GTMP	Global Trachoma Mapping Project
GP	Gram Panchayat
GIA	Grant-In-Aid
HRT	Heidelberg Retinal Tomography
IRR	Incidence Rate Ratio
ICER	Incremental Cost-Effectiveness Ratio
ICMR	Indian Council of Medical Research
IPHS	Indian Public Health Standards
IEC	Information, Education, and Communication
ICDS	Integrated Child Development Services
IAPB	International Agency for The Prevention of Blindness
ICD	International Classification of Disease
ICF	International Classification of Functioning, Disability, and Health Impairments
ICIDH-I	International Classification of Impairments, Disabilities, and Handicaps
ISGEO	International Society for Geographic and Epidemiologic Ophthalmology
IOL	Intraocular Lens
IOP	Intraocular Pressure
LOCS	Lens Opacities Classification System
LFU	Lost to Follow-Up
LVR	Low-Vision Rehabilitation
MAS	Mahila Arogya Samitis
MIS	Management Information System

MRN	Medical Record Number
MGD	Meibomian Gland Dysfunction
MLHP	Mid-Level Health Provider
MLP	Mid-Level Personnel
MOH&FW	Ministry of Health and Family Welfare
MAR	Missing at Random
MCAR	Missing Completely at Random
MSVI	Moderate Severe Visual Impairment
MVI	Moderate Visual Impairment
MTS	Multi-Tasking Staff
MDMOU	Multipurpose District Mobile Ophthalmic Units
NBVI	National Blindness and Visual Impairment Survey
NHM	National Health Mission
NPCB&VI	National Programme for Control of Blindness and Visual Impairment
NSC	National Screening Committee
NRM	Natural Resource Management
NPV	Net Present Value
NCD	Non-Communicable Disease
NGOS	Non-Governmental Organizations
NIM	North India Myopia
NE	North-Eastern
NMAR	Not Missing at Random
NC	Nuclear Colour
NO	Nuclear Opalescence
OHTS	Ocular Hypertension Treatment Study
OR	Odds Ratio
ODK	Open Data Kit
OT	Operation Theatre
OCT	Optical Coherence Tomography
PRI	Panchayati Raj Institutions
PMOA	Paramedical Ophthalmic Assistant
POL	Petroleum, Oil, and Lubricants
PAR	Population Attributable Risk
PCO	Posterior Capsular Opacification
P	Posterior Subcapsular Zone
PMJAY	Pradhan Mantri Jan Arogya Yojana
PV	Present Value
PVA	Presenting Visual Acuity
PAC	Primary Angle Closure
PACG	Primary Angle-Closure Glaucoma
PEC	Primary Eye Care
PHC	Primary Health Centre
POAG	Primary Open-Angle Glaucoma
PSU	Primary Sampling Units
PPS	Probability Proportional to Size
PIP	Programme Implementation Plan

PPP	Public–Private Partnerships
QALY	Quality-Adjusted Life Years
RCT	Randomized Control Trial
RAAB	Rapid Assessment of Avoidable Blindness
RACSS	Rapid Assessment of Cataract Surgical Services
RAVI	Rapid Assessment of Visual Impairment
RATA	Rapid Assistive Technology Assessment
RE	Refractive Errors
RIO	Regional Institutes of Ophthalmology
RP	Retinitis Pigmentosa
ROP	Retinopathy of Prematurity
SNDREAMS	Sankara Nethralaya Diabetic Retinopathy Epidemiology and Molecular Genetics Study
SHG	Self-Help Groups
SVI	Severe Visual Impairment
SRS	Simple Random Sampling
SPSS	Statistical Package for Social Sciences
SC	Sub-Centre
SHC	Sub-Health Centres
SDH	Sub-District Hospital
SDG	Sustainable Development Goals
TCO	Trachomatous Corneal Opacity
TT	Trachomatous Trichiasis
UV	Ultraviolet
UIN	Unique Identification Number
UHC	Universal Health Coverage
ULB	Urban Local Bodies
VC	Vision Centre
VA	Visual Acuity
VI	Visual Impairment
VAD	Vitamin A Deficiency
WHA	World Health Assembly
WHO	World Health Organization
WHO CHOICE	World Health Organization Choosing Interventions that are Cost-Effective

1

Concepts of Community Ophthalmology (Public Health for Eye Care)

G. V. S. MURTHY

1.1 GENESIS OF PUBLIC HEALTH AND PUBLIC HEALTH FOR EYE CARE/COMMUNITY OPHTHALMOLOGY

Though not called public health, activities contributing to improved health of populations have been in practice since time immemorial. Ancient communities in Babylon, China, Peru, Mexico, and India (1) laid emphasis on sanitation and clean drinking water, used medicinal plants, and practiced effective surgery, suturing, fumigation, personal hygiene, diet, and exercise. Over time, it was realized that ensuring the health of populations was not the prerogative of only the governments, but that civil society also had a role to play. This led to the development of community health, where multiple stakeholders partnered to drive success.

Eye conditions and their management have also been known for generations. Trachoma is one of the earliest known diseases of mankind. It was known to ancient Chinese physicians in 2700 BC, and in Egypt around 2000 BC. Babylonian and Vedic literature of 2000 BC aptly describes cataract and its treatment. Sushruta and Ashwini Kumar practiced couching before the advent of the Christian era (2). Couching is believed to have originated in India. From India, the technique spread to Alexandria and later was accepted in West Africa. Vision screening of schoolchildren began in 1867 in Europe, and such programmes were initiated in America in 1894.

The prevention of ophthalmia neonatorum also engaged the attention of physicians of the colonies. Crede's method of prophylaxis using silver nitrate was introduced in 1880.

DOI: 10.1201/9781003291626-1

The application of epidemiological principles to the practice of ophthalmology is half a century old. Norman Gregg and S. H. Clifford were pioneers in this area. The relationship between rubella and congenital cataracts was first observed by Gregg. In 1941, a paediatrician contributed significantly to ophthalmic knowledge. In Boston, S. H. Clifford noted unusual opacities in the eyes of a premature infant; within a week, he saw a second case and then began the "epidemic" of retrolental fibroplasia, and it took 10,000 children before the practice of excess oxygen could be pinpointed and stopped.

Community-based programmes have always interested the ophthalmic fraternity. Sir Henry Holland instituted the first eye camp in India in the 19th century. India and Pakistan continued with the tradition of serving the populations bereft of eye surgeons through the modicum of eye camps. In the 1950s, a large amount of work was conducted to find a suitable method for mass treatment of trachoma. Five decades ago, India also experimented successfully with mass treatment using topical tetracycline eye ointment.

In dealing with eye morbidity and visual loss, two distinct approaches are in practice:

- An individual-based clinical care model where care is provided at the facility level.
- A community-based/population-based approach which looks at improving access to people in a population needing care and modalities to prevent eye ill health and improve productivity by instituting measures at the population level. This domain of care falls in the realm of community ophthalmology/public health for eye care.

1.2 WHAT IS COMMUNITY OPHTHALMOLOGY?

Community ophthalmology, also known as public health for eye care or community eye care, is the application of principles of public health and community health in the field of eye care. It therefore embodies an all-encompassing multidisciplinary approach that goes beyond clinical ophthalmology to improve or preserve the "sense" of vision that is so critical to quality of life and well-being of individuals and communities. Community ophthalmology therefore builds on the gains of clinical ophthalmology.

To understand the concept of community ophthalmology, it is important to look at the continuum of vision or ocular health on the one hand and the underlying causation of disease, including the social determinants, on the other. Ocular health is a continuum from the "ideal" of being able to see at a distance and near without any aids or appliances (spectacles, low-vision aids, vision-restoring cataract surgery, anti-VEGF for diabetic retinopathy, etc.) or any abnormalities of the eye to the other extreme of the spectrum, where vision is lost (Figure 1.1).

Unlike clinical interventions like a cataract surgery or laser for ROP or anti-VEGF for diabetic retinopathy, where the clinical outcomes are tangible and seen

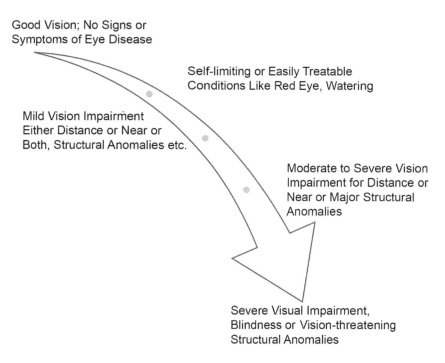

Good Vision; No Signs or Symptoms of Eye Disease

Self-limiting or Easily Treatable Conditions Like Red Eye, Watering

Mild Vision Impairment Either Distance or Near or Both, Structural Anomalies etc.

Moderate to Severe Vision Impairment for Distance or Near or Major Structural Anomalies

Severe Visual Impairment, Blindness or Vision-threatening Structural Anomalies

Figure 1.1 Continuum of vision loss and structural anomalies.

immediately, in community ophthalmology/public health for eye care, the benefits are not immediately perceived and may take a long time to be measured—for example, reduction in blindness prevalence in a region or equitable access for women to phacoemulsification cataract surgery as men.

1.3 DEFINING COMMUNITY OPHTHALMOLOGY

Community ophthalmology can be aptly defined as collective action for sustained population-wide equitable, affordable, and quality eye health outcomes. Formal health systems are the drivers of community ophthalmology, as they have the bandwidth and capacity to fund and sustain efforts in the long run.

When a mother breastfeeds her child immediately after delivery, it is a personal achievement for that mother-and-child unit, but when the messaging on need for breastfeeding immediately after birth is popularized by the government or 75% of mothers in a population breastfeed their babies within the first hour of birth, that is public health success. Collective action needs authority and accountability of large population groups. The government usually has administrative authority and the legal support to make things happen by coordinating and directing the efforts of all those involved in improving health.

Community ophthalmology owes its existence to public health and ophthalmology. Therefore, community ophthalmology practice uses skills from both these major disciplines. The underlying principle in public health is organized community effort to improve health outcomes. The same applied to improve eye health outcomes translates into community ophthalmology or public health for eye care. Community ophthalmology is therefore primarily concerned with identifying and studying the distribution (magnitude) and determinants (causes) of eye diseases and vision status of populations so as to facilitate planning, implementation, and evaluation of a set of strategies to improve vision status and functioning of people within the population and the assessment of whether population needs have been met or not.

The broad goal of community ophthalmology is to reduce ocular ill health and vision loss, with a mission of promoting quality of life.

Community ophthalmology denotes the use of appropriate strategies to reduce the burden of eye disease in the community, and the consequences of ocular ill health, while striving to ensure the best possible ocular health status for a major proportion of the community. In other words, *community ophthalmology* can be defined as the use of the full scope of ophthalmic and public health knowledge, skills, and services to promote the ocular health of groups of people, particularly at community level, thereby directly improving the quality of life of individuals, families, and communities.

Community ophthalmology practice therefore signifies the promotion of good ocular health, the prevention of ocular morbidity and disability, the treatment of curable blindness, and rehabilitation of the incurably blind. The parameters for measuring success of this approach of preservation, promotion, and insulation against ocular disease and disability are in terms of what proportion of the population has benefited from the interventions canvassed.

Absolute numbers and individual visual improvement are monitored in clinical ophthalmology practice, while in community ophthalmology/public health for eye care, the "denominator" is crucial. The "denominator" is either the whole population or the population at risk or an appropriate segment, such as children, elderly, men, women, rural residents, urban dwellers, etc. The "numerator" is the number of people who received a service or benefitted from a service. This allows programme managers to identify what proportion of the population was covered and what is the quantum of work that needs to be completed. The denominator also allows comparisons across regions or countries. Without an appropriate denominator, the measurement of success of any programmatic intervention is not possible.

A frequently asked question is that if both in clinical as well as in community practice clinical services are ultimately provided to individuals, how do the two approaches differ? The difference is in the unit of interest in the two approaches. In clinical practice, the focus of interest is the benefit to the treated individual, while in public health for eye care practice, the spotlight is on how much difference an intervention led to. To illustrate the point, an ophthalmologist in an eye hospital is professionally satisfied that they have operated three retinal detachments, two trabeculectomies, and five cataracts in a week and all the patients recovered well. But in community ophthalmology practice, the "pundits" are happy with the ten surgeries but are not completely "satisfied" as millions are still awaiting their turn to see light at the end of the tunnel.

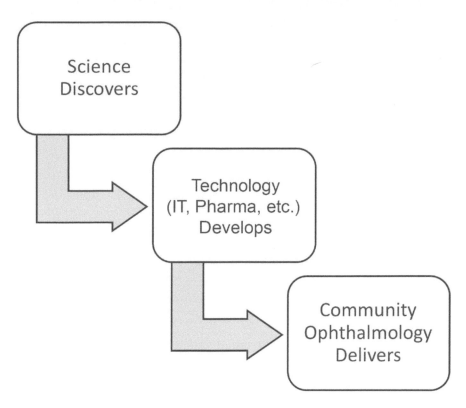

Figure 1.2 From the laboratory to the population.

Community ophthalmology ensures that what is discovered by research is further developed and contextualized by technology before being offered at the community level (Figure 1.2). Since community ophthalmology targets big population groups and communities, any intervention or service delivered at this level has to be backed by strong scientific evidence. Therefore, evidence-based practice, which is the process of integrating science-based interventions with the preferences of the communities to improve the health of populations (3), is of critical importance to the practice of community ophthalmology.

1.4 CORE FUNCTIONS AND CHARACTERISTICS

The core functions of community ophthalmology are illustrated in Figure 1.3.

Without authority for action, the different partners in a coalition cannot achieve results. Therefore, for public health efforts to succeed, the government is the fulcrum towards which all other partners gravitate.

Public health for eye care/community ophthalmology therefore strives for accessibility, availability, affordability, and appropriateness of services for all while ensuring accountability of the health system to achieve quality of care.

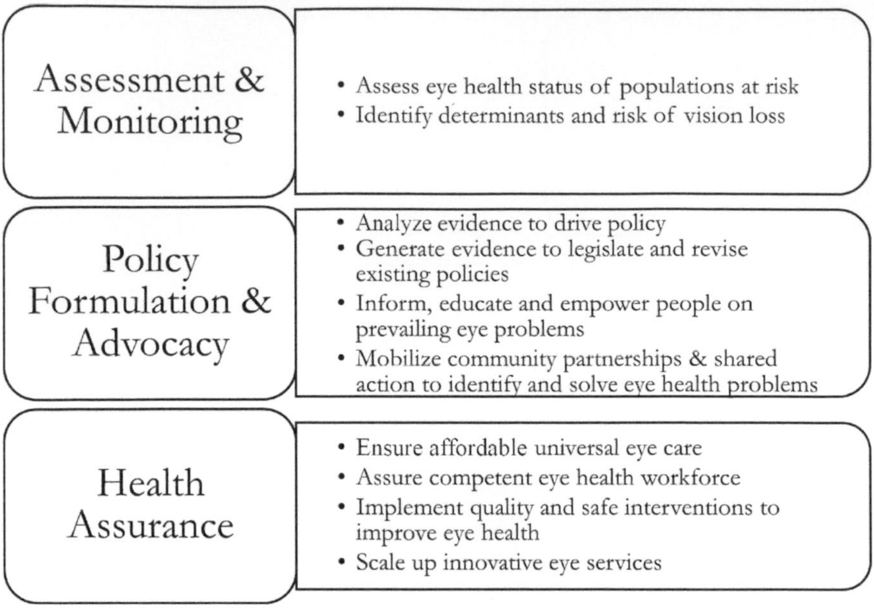

Assessment & Monitoring	• Assess eye health status of populations at risk • Identify determinants and risk of vision loss
Policy Formulation & Advocacy	• Analyze evidence to drive policy • Generate evidence to legislate and revise existing policies • Inform, educate and empower people on prevailing eye problems • Mobilize community partnerships & shared action to identify and solve eye health problems
Health Assurance	• Ensure affordable universal eye care • Assure competent eye health workforce • Implement quality and safe interventions to improve eye health • Scale up innovative eye services

Figure 1.3 Core functions of community ophthalmology.

The functions of community ophthalmology/public health for eye care are therefore manifold (Figure 1.4).

1.5 CHARACTERISTICS OF COMMUNITY OPHTHALMOLOGY/PUBLIC HEALTH FOR EYE CARE

- The primary focus of community ophthalmology is on population-level interventions to improve eye care.
- The emphasis is on a comprehensive basket of services which include prevention and health promotion.
- The discipline employs a broad spectrum of interventions which target both direct etiopathogenesis of an eye condition as well as the social determinants, especially those that can be modified.
- Community ophthalmology is a shared responsibility of the public health system (government owned), health professionals, and the community.
- It brings together a convergence of multiple professional competencies ranging from clinicians to behavioural scientists, epidemiologists, technologists, and biostatisticians.
- Equity, which includes equality and non-discrimination in the provision of services, access, or equivalence in outcomes, is fundamental to the practice of community ophthalmology.
- The basic premise of community ophthalmology is that whole populations rather than discrete individuals alone benefit from eye care services.

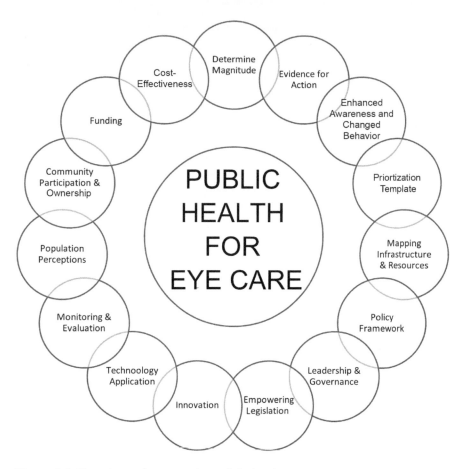

Figure 1.4 Functions of community ophthalmology.

- Community ophthalmology services ensure that all individuals comprising a population have an equal opportunity to attain optimal ocular health within the existing socioeconomic context of a country.
- Community ophthalmology empowers communities to take ownership of service delivery to ensure sustainability of services.
- Improved eye health directly or indirectly contributes to most of the Sustainable Development Goals, and therefore, operationalizing universal eye care as part of universal healthcare is a key tenet of community ophthalmology/public health for eye care. This will ensure both enhanced access to eye services and protection of populations from financial hardship to access needed eye care services.
- Current thinking differentiates between the "biomedical" delivery of health services (the public health systems—the micro-environment) and the macro-environment which promotes health and prevents disease by looking at all factors that impact on health status and health behaviours.

- Community ophthalmology yields rich dividends for population eye health status. Gains are incremental based on the inputs invested in the public health systems.
- Population-based big data analytics, digital technology, epidemiological modelling, and artificial intelligence will be the future face of community ophthalmology as it will cover a large number of people in the shortest possible time and provide more accurate predictions of future trends.

Public health for eye care also recognizes that attaining optimal or best possible health status for populations or individuals within a population is dependent not only on the risk factors or provision of health services alone but also on all sectors of social development which have a direct or indirect impact on health. These "social determinants" include, among others, education, water, sanitation, nutrition, food production, availability and distribution, economically remunerative employment, congenial social relationships. etc. While striving towards achieving the Sustainable Development Goals (SDGs), due attention needs to be paid to the social determinants too (Figure 1.5).

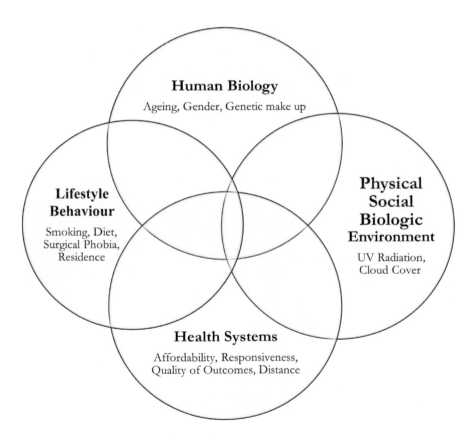

Figure 1.5 Determinants of vision loss.

1.6 COMPARISON OF CLINICAL AND COMMUNITY OPHTHALMOLOGY

The differences between the clinical care and community care approaches are highlighted in Table 1.1.

Table 1.1 Comparison of Community Ophthalmology and Clinical Ophthalmology

Parameters	Clinical Ophthalmology	Community Ophthalmology
Unit of interest	Individuals with an eye problem	Populations residing in specified catchment areas
Diagnostic tools	Clinical examination	Surveys, screening to establish community diagnosis and profile risk groups
Management protocols	Diagnose and treat	Diagnose, treat, prevent
Treatment modalities	Drugs/surgery/appliances/rehabilitation	Health awareness, behaviour change communication, health system strengthening
Measure of success	Patient satisfaction	Population free of an eye disease and improved health
Foundations	Clinical skills	Epidemiology, statistics and management, communication and clinical skills
Evidence generation	Clinical trials, case reports, case control studies	Community intervention trials, observational studies
Domain	"Retail" philosophy, where a small number of individuals are managed	"Wholesale" philosophy, where health is elivered on a scale, with many benefitting from an intervention

1.7 THE NEED FOR COMMUNITY OPHTHALMOLOGY PRACTICE

Most eye ailments can be diagnosed with relative ease and managed effectively by primary care interventions. Eighty percent of ocular problems can either be diagnosed and treated or diagnosed and referred by health auxiliaries. Community ophthalmology practice endeavours to augment the skills of auxiliaries in order to provide comprehensive eye care services. It is not possible to sit in isolated ivory towers in overgrown metropolises and hope that the whole population would benefit by providing purely hospital-based services. One has to venture beyond the four walls if one is to make a dent on ocular ill health.

Most eye diseases are either preventable or easily curable in the early stages. Even 90% of blindness is either preventable or curable. It is abundantly clear that prevention is more cost-effective than cure and long-term rehabilitation. Intervening early mitigates the potential disability and handicap of severe visual impairment and blindness that may occur at a later stage.

The typical pattern of disease encountered in hospitals is not representative of community ill health. Patients come to the hospitals in the late and terminal stages or when they perceive their ailment as sight-threatening. Since most eye diseases in the early stages do not manifest any serious symptoms and develop innocuously, patients tend to ignore them. Thus, the incipient and mild cases will only be seen in the community. Community-based services can bring such cases to the attention of healthcare providers.

Awareness of causality, potential solutions, and accessible eye care facilities are important if people perceive the seriousness of their eye ailment and seek treatment early. Behavioural change communication (BCC) has to be delivered at the population level for improved compliance. This is one of the many facets of community ophthalmology. This will also reduce unnecessary financial stress and catastrophic health expenditures at a later date.

A community intervention is a cost-effective strategy that attempts to prevent disease and promote health by instituting technologically sound and scientifically proven strategies at community level, to the largest number of those in need.

To summarize, community ophthalmology or public health for eye care has pioneering application in low- and middle-income countries like India due to the following reasons:

1. It helps in optimizing the available resources by prioritizing the needs of the many rather than the selected few.
2. To attain sustainable development goals, community ophthalmology can play a vital role.
3. Community ophthalmology can help in early detection and prompt referral and management, thereby reducing costs to the healthcare system.

REFERENCES

1. Singh V. Sushruta: The father of surgery. Natl J Maxillofac Surg 2017; 8(1): 1–3.
2. Kansupada KB, Sassani JW. Sushruta: The father of Indian surgery and ophthalmology. Doc Ophthalmol 1997; 93(1–2): 159–67.
3. Kohatsu ND, Robinson JG, Torner JC. Evidence-based public health: An evolving concept. Am J Prev Med 2004; 27(5): 417–21.

2

Basic Epidemiology, Statistics, and Research Methodology

PRAVEEN VASHIST, SOUVIK MANNA, PALLAVI SHUKLA, VIVEK GUPTA

2.1 DEFINITION AND HISTORICAL EVOLUTION OF EPIDEMIOLOGY

Epidemiology emanates from the Greek work "epi," meaning *upon*; "demo," meaning *population*; and "logy," meaning *study*. Hence, it is the study upon population. One of the first definitions of the term was coined by A. Lilienfeld in 1980: "Epidemiology is concerned with the patterns of disease occurrence in human populations and the factors that influence these patterns" (1). John M. Last has defined *epidemiology* in 2001 as "the study of the distribution and determinants of health-related states or events in specified populations, and the application of this study to control of health problems" (2). This branch has evolved successively over the centuries from an initial focus on infectious disease to non-communicable diseases and, finally, to emerging and re-emerging diseases, especially the Covid-19 pandemic. In terms of eye disease, *epidemiology* can be defined as "the study of patterns of eye diseases in human populations and the determinants of these patterns."

2.2 WHY IS EPIDEMIOLOGY IMPORTANT?

It is important for the following reasons:

1. Epidemiological research contributes to the body of scientific knowledge about diseases of the eye and provides clues to their likely aetiological pathways, which may not emerge from laboratory research or observation in the clinic.

DOI: 10.1201/9781003291626-2

2. It contributes to the public health approach to blindness prevention by identifying the magnitude of the problem and describing the main causes and distribution of eye diseases that result in impairment and disability. It also identifies differences between populations that may be modifiable.
3. Epidemiological research also contributes to blindness prevention through understanding the determinants of disease in human populations.
4. Epidemiology evaluates preventive measures, treatments, or other interventions to reduce the impact of vision loss, by conducting clinical trials that require randomization of populations or persons, together with standardized assessments of outcome (3).

Thus, the epidemiology of eye disease has made, and continues to make, critical contributions to both scientific knowledge and blindness prevention. In this chapter, we review the concepts and principles of ophthalmic epidemiology that are useful for effective control of eye diseases.

2.3 THE EVOLUTION OF OPHTHALMIC EPIDEMIOLOGY

Rapid Assessment of Cataract Surgical Services (RACSS) was the initial methodology for the study of ophthalmic epidemiology, with special focus on cataract. While still being population-based, rapid assessment techniques have also been improved over the last 15 years. Employed initially for assessment of cataract blindness (RACSS), these methods are now being increasingly used for gathering evidence of other causes of visual impairment (VI), both at local and national level. The Rapid Assessment of Avoidable Blindness (RAAB), Rapid Assessment of Visual Impairment (RAVI), and Rapid Assistive Technology Assessment (rATA) are all new methods to study diverse components of the epidemiology of the eye (4, 5). The definitions of blindness and visual impairment have also been modified by WHO from those based on best corrected visual acuity (BCVA) to presenting visual acuity (PVA) (6). Evidence on the extent of the problem and the magnitude of refractive errors (REs) can only be collected if the definition of blindness and VI includes uncorrected and under-corrected REs. Most surveys in the late 1990s and the first two decades of the 21st century have therefore used presenting or habitual vision, a cut-off level of 6/12 for visual impairment and near vision testing along with distance vision. The introduction of pinhole vision testing also allows an estimate of refractive errors.

A series of surveys, covering the population aged 50 years and above, has been conducted over the period of 1998–2019. Though they have used different protocols of examination (RACSS, comprehensive, or RAAB), the data can be compared with respect to presenting visual acuity. Despite all the limitations of the comparisons, it is evident that there has been an appreciable change during the period of 1998–2019, which was a significant decrease in the prevalence of blindness from 5.3% to 1.99% in population aged 50 years and above for PVA <3/60 in better eye.

2.4 PATTERNS OF DISTRIBUTION OF BLINDNESS

Demography. The overall prevalence of blindness is a function of age, affecting mainly the older section of any population. Over the previous 12–18 years, the estimated prevalence of global blindness has risen more or less in step with the increase in world population. However, the number of people in the group aged 25–40 years has been larger than in earlier age strata. As this works its way into the older age bands in around 20 years' time, the prevalence of blindness will be expected to rise at a faster rate than the total population, if appropriate interventions are not put in place.

A meta-analysis has been completed to show the influence of gender on blindness (7). It showed that, globally, women bear excess blindness compared to men. The excess of blindness in women was marked among the elderly and not only due to differential life expectancy. The excess burden of blindness among women is likely due to a number of factors, including less access to family financial resources, requirement of assistance to travel with fewer options to travel, as well as lack of access to information. These factors may be different in industrialized countries as compared to developing countries.

Geography. The prevalence of diseases like trachoma depends on geography even within the same country. Trachoma is endemic in the northern and western arid areas of India, whereas it is unheard of in the eastern and north-eastern region. Even the cases in the southern states are unlikely to be caused by local transmission, as the environmental characteristics of the south are not conducive to chlamydial growth and transmission.

Literacy. Data from National Blindness Survey India and from many other countries have shown that literacy is one of the most important determinants of the prevalence of blindness. According to the NPCB&VI (2015–2019) survey, illiterate rural females were the most affected with blindness.

2.5 STUDY DESIGNS IN EPIDEMIOLOGY

The diversity of methods used in epidemiological research may be grouped into two primary types (Figure 2.1)

Randomized experimental studies. The gold standard of randomized experimental studies is the RCT. In this type of study, the researchers randomly allocate participants to "exposure" (therapeutic or preventive intervention) or not (control). The "unexposed" or control group may receive nothing, a placebo, or the standard treatment. Allocation is random so that if the groups are sufficiently large, they should be similar with respect to all extraneous factors, known and unknown, which might influence the outcome. For instance, they will be similar in terms of age structure, health conditions, and body size. This means that any difference in outcome between the comparison groups could be attributed to the exposure to "treatment" under study rather than any other difference between the two groups. The intervention and control groups are then followed over time to assess disease incidence; the incidence in the intervention group is compared with

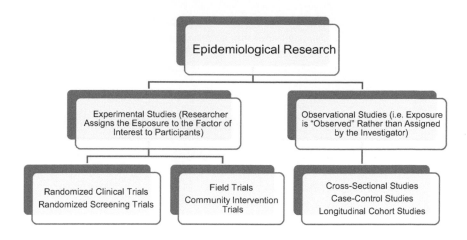

Figure 2.1 Study designs in epidemiology.

that in the control group to assess the effect of the intervention on the disease risk. Participants and researchers are typically masked to the exposure status of the participants, meaning, that they do not know to which group the participant has been assigned, and this is done in order to reduce bias in reporting and assessment of disease. As an example, an RCT was done in Delhi to compare the efficacy of physiological, non-detergent eyelid wipes with conventional lid hygiene in patients with meibomian gland dysfunction (MGD) (8). Significant improvement in symptoms and signs of MGD was observed in the eyelid wipes group, which was maintained even after adjusting for sociodemographic variables, such as age, sex, and severity score of symptoms and signs.

Variants on the RCT model exist, such as the randomized screening trial. Another variant is the field trial, where individuals in a population are randomized to a preventive intervention (e.g. a vaccine) or no intervention (or placebo) and the incidence of disease compared in the two groups. Such trials have been used for diseases that are of great public health concern. Some of the largest experimental studies have been of this type, for example, the Salk vaccine trial for poliomyelitis, involving more than one million children.

Community intervention trials. They are similar to field trials, but in this design, convenient clusters of people (communities) rather than individuals are randomized to the preventive intervention. An example is the first community-based vitamin A trial (9).

The main limitations of randomized experimental studies arise from two sources. First, for practical reasons, strict eligibility criteria have to be used in the selection of subjects so that the observations are often made on a highly selected sample. Consequently, the inferences may be limited to small, and sometimes peculiar, populations rather than to a large population of general interest. Secondly, randomization may be unethical if one of the interventions or treatments is regarded to be more beneficial by clinicians or by the patients. Moreover, it may not be feasible to randomize exposure to certain biological, behavioural, or other psychosocial factors (e.g. smoking, stress, or alcoholism). The high cost of experimental studies in some situations is an additional disadvantage. In view of these limitations, most epidemiological investigations of aetiological factors are observational in design.

2.6 OBSERVATIONAL STUDIES: BASIC DESIGNS

In observational studies, the investigators observe the events as they unfold naturally. There are three main basic types of observational study.

Cross-sectional surveys. In a cross-sectional study, the investigators carefully sample people from the population. They then examine and/or interview the participants to assess whether or not they have the disease and exposure(s) of interest. This allows assessment of the prevalence of disease (and exposure) so that the magnitude of disease in the population can be estimated. The prevalence can also be compared in different groups (e.g. those exposed and those unexposed) to explore whether there may be an association between the exposure and the disease. As an example, in the national blindness survey conducted in India, the overall prevalence of blindness in population aged 50+ years was 1.99% (95% CI: 1.94–2.13) (10). However, with cross-sectional surveys, we must emphasize the adage that "association does not equal causation." We do not know whether the exposure or disease came first, or if both are caused by a third factor.

They are also known as population-based sample surveys. The only secure source of prevalence data are population-based prevalence surveys conducted according to strict criteria. Because data are now available from a large number of surveys, it becomes important to identify those which can stand the test of scientific rigour. In this chapter, we have required some basic criteria, as follows:

1. The survey must have identified the population to which it refers and selected a sample using random sampling methods so that the results can be generalized to the wider population in that area.
2. If it is to be generalizable, the survey should include a representative population and not be limited only to specific groups in, for example, areas endemic for trachoma, leprosy villages. This will allow the findings to be extrapolated to a wider population.
3. A sample should be large enough to provide confidence intervals (95%) on the prevalence measures. If blindness is relatively rare, the estimate will be un-interpretable, unless the sample size is large.
4. Clear-cut descriptions should be provided of the sampling process, definition used, enumeration procedure adopted, clinical examination protocol followed, and methods of data analysis.

Establishing an association between exposure to a risk factor or causative agent and the presence or absence of disease requires an analytical study design. This may either be a case-control study or a longitudinal (cohort) study, which may, in turn, be retrospective or prospective.

Cohort studies. Cohort studies allow us to measure disease incidence rather than focusing on prevalence, as in the cross-sectional studies. To conduct a cohort study, a group of people free from the disease of interest is selected (i.e. prevalent cases are excluded). The participants are then examined or interviewed and are categorized as "exposed" or "unexposed" with respect to the risk factor of interest. The participants are then followed over time, and the number of incident cases of disease that arise is assessed. This allows the investigators to calculate the incidence of disease (whether cumulative incidence or incidence rate). The incidence can be calculated separately in the exposed and unexposed group so that the relative risk can be estimated.

The North India myopia (NIM) study was a longitudinal cohort study of 10,000 schoolchildren aged 5 to 15 years who were followed up for an interval of one year to identify new myopes (spherical equivalent $\leq$ -0.5D) and progression of myopia in previously diagnosed myopic children (11). Out of the 9,616 children re-screened (97.3% coverage), annual incidence of myopia was 3.4%, and progression was observed in 49.2% of the children. There was a significant higher incidence of myopia in younger children compared to older children (P = 0.012) and among girls compared to boys (P = 0.002) (11).

This example illustrates the problem of loss to follow-up, which is often encountered by cohort studies. Not all the initial cohort were included in the final analyses, and it is not known what happened to those lost to follow-up in terms of myopia. This means that the risk measured may not be "true" risk in that study population. Another problem with cohort studies is that they usually require either a large sample or long follow-up to accumulate enough incident cases of disease to have sufficient power to make meaningful inferences. This makes cohort studies expensive and time-consuming, which is why they are rare in the ophthalmic literature. The strengths of cohort studies are that incidence can be estimated and that the researchers are relatively confident that the exposure preceded the disease.

2.7 CASE-CONTROL STUDIES

They are used to study the aetiology of disease and are conducted by recruiting people who have the disease of interest (cases) as well as people without the disease (controls) to allow comparison. The cases and controls are then interviewed or examined to assess whether they have the exposure of interest. The odds of being exposed are then compared for cases and controls to see if there is an association between exposure and being a case. Ideally, cases are "incident cases" so that they are newly diagnosed and have not had time to change their exposure status as a result of their diagnosis. The controls are selected from the same population that gave rise to the cases and represent the exposure distribution in the source population. Case control cannot be used to estimate the burden of disease, since the ratio of cases to controls is determined by the investigators.

A case-control study was done to determine the effect of exposure to high level of air pollution in Delhi on ocular surface health, in which a total of 520 subjects volunteered to participate (12). A significantly high number of subjects in study group complained of ophthalmic symptoms compared to the control group; 78% of the subjects in the study group had symptoms such as redness, watering, irritation, strain, or photophobia, whereas this number was 45% in the control group. These results suggest that in Delhi there is an association between high levels of pollution and having ocular surface disease.

There are many advantages to case-control studies. They are relatively quick and cheap to carry out and can be used to investigate rare diseases. Recall bias is a problem since cases and controls may report exposure history differently because of their case status. Avoiding bias due to selection of inappropriate controls is also a major challenge.

Nested case-control studies. They combine some of the advantageous features of case-control and cohort studies. For example, in one common form, all disease cases occurring in a given population are identified through a registry. A sample of non-cases (sometimes matched for age, etc.) is also drawn from the same population. The past exposure status is then ascertained for both the cases and the sample of non-cases. Here, the number of non-cases that has to be investigated for past exposure is only a small fraction of the numbers in a longitudinal cohort study (particularly when the disease is rare). An important advantage over a case-control study design is that a measure of disease frequency can be estimated for the population.

Ecological studies. In the ecological study design, the exposure status data are not available for individuals but are obtained as an average for groups. The unit of observation is thus the group rather than an individual. The groups are commonly defined geographically (e.g. as a whole country or region) but could be defined by other factors, such as socioeconomic, occupational, and demographic factors. A proxy measure is often used to describe the exposure status of the group, as individual measures are not obtained. For instance, average per capita gross domestic product for the country could be used as the measure of socioeconomic status. Comparisons are made between the groups in respect to frequency of disease occurrence. Examples include a study to measure association between cataract and sun exposure along with other environmental risk factors in three different geographically diverse populations of rural India from 2010 to 2016 (13). The three different areas include plain area in the north (Gurugram), hilly area in the northeast (Guwahati), and coastal area in the south (Prakasam). The various geographical zones were defined according to average levels of ambient ultraviolet radiation and were then compared with respect to the population prevalence of cataract. It is now well-known that inferences from ecological data may be misleading. The problem, named "ecologic fallacy," arises because there are often insufficient data on other pertinent exposures to allow control of confounding in the analysis. In addition, the exposure and disease status of individuals are not known, and so even if an association between the exposure and disease exists at the population level, it may not exist at the individual level.

Self-controlled case series. It can be used to assess the effect of a transient exposure on disease risk. A patient who has developed a disease is interviewed about his/her exposure pattern during a specific period of time. This time is divided into "risk" periods and "control" periods. For instance, imagine that an investigator wishes to assess the relationship between the administration of dilatation drops and the development of acute open-angle glaucoma. The investigator would interview cases of acute open-angle glaucoma about whether or not they had received dilatation drops during the 24 hours prior to disease onset. The period in the two hours before disease onset could be defined as the "risk" period, while the previous 22 hours are the "control" period. The investigator can then assess whether the onset of disease is associated with the administration of drops. This study design includes only cases, and the cases act as their own controls; therefore, any potential association between the exposure and disease cannot be attributed to differences in age or other risk factors (i.e. confounding is removed).

Space/time cluster studies. They share the features of ecological studies insofar as exposure data are not available for individuals and clusters or groups are compared. In addition, the grouping need not be according to levels of exposure to a particular putative risk factor. The studies are designed to detect clustering in space, that is, a non-uniform distribution of "cases" over the total study area, beyond the level of clustering that might be expected from the population distribution and chance. The studies have been used to implicate or assess general environmental influences in the disease aetiology. Examples include international comparisons of disease risk or prevalence.

Time clustering studies are designed to detect non-uniform distribution of the occurrence of cases over a time period for a defined population. The main objectives are to identify secular trends in large populations, including cyclic fluctuations, and to explore local epidemics. Time clustering designs are sometimes combined with space clustering designs to detect clustering in time and space. Clustering of cases in both time and space suggests the involvement of infectious agents in causation of the disease.

Genetic studies. There is enormous interest in identifying genetic risk factors for disease. This can be investigated through cross-sectional surveys, cohort studies, or case-control studies by including genotype as the exposure and assessing its role in the aetiology of disease. There are also specific study designs used for genetic studies: twin studies, familial aggregation studies, and pedigree studies.

2.8 MEASUREMENT OF FREQUENCY OF EYE DISEASES

2.8.1 Definition: Magnitude

Magnitude is the size of the problem of a condition or disease. The two measures used are prevalence and incidence. *Prevalence* is a static measure that provides a snapshot of the disease in the population at a particular point in time and includes all cases of disease regardless of duration.

Prevalence is a proportion and relates to a defined population:

$$Prevalence = \frac{number\ of\ cases\ of\ disease\ at\ a\ particular\ time}{total\ number\ of\ the\ population}$$

This crude prevalence measure can be made more specific by giving the prevalence in a particular age group—for example, the number of people with blindness aged 50–59 years as a proportion of the total defined population aged 50–59 years. This is called the age-specific prevalence. For meaningful comparison between studies in different populations, or in the same population at different times, prevalence can be adjusted to a reference population with a known age and sex structure.

The results of many published surveys are expressed as single figures. The prevalence is, however, an estimate, the accuracy of which depends on total numbers examined and on the sampling method. A simple random sample is usually impractical for a national or even district population. Most surveys are therefore based on cluster sampling, the population often having first been stratified.

Incidence is a more dynamic measure of the magnitude of the problem and measures the number of new cases of disease in the population at risk (that is, the population that does not already have the disease) over a defined period of time. Incidence can be expressed in two main ways: either as a proportion or as a rate. Incidence expressed in the simplest way, as a proportion, is known as cumulative incidence (CI).

$$CI = \frac{number\ of\ new\ cases\ occurring\ in\ a\ given\ time}{total\ number\ of\ population\ at\ risk\ at\ the\ beginning\ of\ the\ period}$$

There are two main measures of incidence, described in detail in the following: cumulative incidence (which is the proportion of the population that is disease-free at baseline that develops a disease over a given time period) and incidence density, or incidence rate (which is the number of cases that occur in the population per unit of person-time at risk and is a rate as it has a time dimension).

2.8.2 Incidence of Blindness

Because of the paucity of data, Podgor, Leske, and Ederer developed a formula, based originally on the Framingham results, to calculate incidence from age-specific prevalence for the major conditions causing blindness (14). Until recently, there was virtually no direct measurement of the incidence of blindness, that is, the number of new cases of blindness in a defined population in one year. Two longitudinal follow-up studies in industrialized countries were completed in the 1990s. The surviving persons in the original population-based cohort in Beaver Dam, WI, USA, who were aged 43–86 years at the baseline in 1990, were re-examined after five years and after ten years (15). Similarly, in the Blue Mountains Eye Study, 2,335 persons were available for follow-up at five years (16).

2.9 MEASURES OF EFFECT

Attributable risk. Let us consider the comparison of two risks R_0 and R_1, where R_0 is a baseline risk in those not exposed (or least exposed) to the factor of interest, and R_1 is the risk in those exposed. To calculate the risk among the exposed and unexposed, we can simply calculate the difference $R_1 - R_0$, which is an absolute measure of effect, commonly called attributable risk (AR). From a public health perspective, the magnitude of AR indicates the amount of risk in the exposed group that could be avoided if the group became unexposed, assuming the putative factor is responsible for the difference. A large AR, however, may simply reflect a large R_0 and R_1. Similarly, a small AR may arise when R_0 and R_1 are small, even when R_1 is several times larger than R_0. Thus, the AR is not a good measure of the strength of association between an exposure and a disease in the context of aetiological research.

Relative risk. The natural solution to estimating the association between an exposure and a disease is to calculate a relative measure that is independent of the magnitude of R_0. In epidemiological studies, the most common relative measure is the relative risk, or R_1/R_0. This can also be called the risk ratio, rate ratio, odds ratio, or incidence rate ratio (when R_0 and R_1 are incidence density measure). Relative risk is a good indicator of the strength of association; for example, a value of 1.0 (or close to unity) indicates no association, 2.0 suggests doubling of risk in the exposed, and 0.5 may indicate halving of the risk in the exposed. It is also possible to calculate the prevalence ratio, by dividing the prevalence of diseased in the exposed group by the prevalence in the unexposed group.

Population attributable risk (PAR). A population is made up of people who are exposed and those who are unexposed, and these people may have a different risk of disease. The risk in the total population is therefore determined by the risk in those who are exposed and those who are unexposed (i.e. the prevalence of exposure). Although a large relative risk may indicate that the exposure is of aetiological importance, this does not necessarily mean that the exposure is of public health concern, for example, when the disease or the exposure is extremely rare. For a holistic appreciation of the importance of an exposure (detrimental or beneficial) at the population level, it is necessary to quantify both relative risk and one of its derivatives. PAR (%) gives the proportion of all "cases" (occurring in a general population) that is attributable to the exposure, by subtracting the risk in the unexposed groups from the risk in the total population. That is:

$$Population\,attributable\,risk\,percent\left(PAR\%\right) = \frac{R\left(total\right) - R0}{R\left(total\right)} \times 100$$

For example, if PAR is 3%, it suggests that 3% of the disease could be avoided if risk factor is eliminated from the population. This has meaning only when a causal relationship is assumed between a detrimental exposure and the "case" status. Another form of the equation (which is mathematically the same as the preceding), provided by Miettinen (17), shows the relation between PAR% and RR: PAR% = P(RR − 1)/RR, where *P* is the prevalence (%) of exposure among the "cases."

The utility of PAR% is clear insofar as it gives an impression of the amount of the disease problem that might "disappear" if exposure to the risk factor at issue is removed. This could be valuable in the planning of a preventive intervention.

2.10 ODDS RATIO (OR)

When separate estimates for R_1 and R_0 cannot be made (e.g. in case-control studies), the risk ratio or rate ratio cannot be estimated directly. Usually, in such situations, the study design ordains that a sample of "cases" (individuals with the disease or condition of interest) is obtained and compared with a contemporaneous sample of non-cases. In the simplest form, the data from such studies may be summarized in a 2-by-2 contingency table.

The odds of being "exposed" can be computed for the cases and the non-cases as a/b and c/d, respectively. The exposure odds ratio (OR) is expressed as:

$$OR = \frac{\left(\dfrac{a}{b}\right)}{\left(\dfrac{c}{d}\right)} = \frac{ad}{bc}$$

The OR obtained from well-designed case-control studies is generally believed to give a good indirect estimate of incidence rate ratio (IRR), particularly when the incidence of the "case" status is low (e.g. for rare disease). Regardless of its validity as an indirect measure of IRR, the OR remains a valid measure of the strength of association between exposure and "case" status. Like IRR, greater deviations from unity indicate stronger associations. The OR has become a very popular choice, even when direct estimation of IRR may be possible, due to the ready availability of robust statistical procedures for OR analysis, such as the logistic regression

Table 2.1 Summary of Data (Simplest Form) from a Case-Control or Cross-Sectional Study

Exposure	Cases	Non-Cases	Total
Exposed	a	b	a + b
Non-exposed	c	d	c + d
	a + c	b + d	a + b + c + d

Note: Individuals are classified according to disease status (cases and non-cases) and also by status of exposure to the factor of interest. The cell frequencies are denoted by the letters *a*, *b*, *c*, and *d*.

model. Thus, the OR is frequently used in the analysis of data that come not only from case-control studies but also from clinical trials and from cross-sectional (prevalence data).

2.11 SCREENING OF EYE DISEASE

Preventing disease is vital to secure health. Prevention can be broken down into three separate approaches: primary (preventing occurrence of disease), secondary (preventing the effects of disease), and tertiary (restoring function lost as a results of disease). Screening is an important weapon in the armoury of secondary prevention.

Screening exposes many healthy individuals to an examination to identify a few who may have disease. Clear thinking and a careful evaluation are essential when any screening programme is undertaken. An understanding of the principles of screening and how they apply to the specific condition targeted is mandatory.

Definition:

> Screening is a process of identifying apparently healthy people who may be at increased risk of a disease or condition. They can then be offered information, further tests and appropriate treatment to reduce their risk and/or any complications arising from the disease or condition.
>
> (18)

If the presence of the condition is confirmed, then effective treatment should lead to a better outcome than that associated with presentation later in the clinical course of the disease (when it has become symptomatic). Such an improved outcome may impinge not just on the individual but also on his/her immediate associates or on the population as a whole (e.g. identifying and treating people for DR reduces the cost of blindness to society).

Screening is a public health intervention intended to reduce the population burden of a condition or its consequences. It is often confused with opportunistic testing, sometimes termed *case finding*, when a screening test may be used. An example of case finding is the routine testing of IOP among people presenting with an eye problem other than glaucoma. Opportunistic case finding occurs when a test is offered to an individual without symptoms of the disease when he/she presents to a healthcare practitioner for reasons unrelated to that disease. A population-based screening programme is an organized integrated process where all activities along with screening pathway are planned, coordinated, monitored, and evaluated through a quality assurance framework. All these activities must be resourced adequately to ensure benefits are maximized.

It is now well recognized that effects of screening may not always be beneficial and that harmful outcomes can occur. These arise as a result of errors of the screening test: mistaken designation as being disease-free or affected (i.e. both false-negative and false-positive test results) that can have serious consequences. The test itself may also potentially be harmful.

An important consideration of screening is that it is a health intervention imposed on the population and so has important ethical implications. Traditionally, medical care is provided for those who seek help. Screening aims to provide healthcare before help is sought in order to identify and treat illness at an earlier stage in its natural history and thereby achieve a better outcome. Individuals must not be coerced, yet their participation is essential if the programme is to be effective. This can only be achieved by convincing the public that being screened offers real benefits to the individual or the community. The benefits must be tangible and well understood by the public without causing undue alarm or anxiety.

Public anxiety can be allayed in part through a robust quality assurance process. This ensures that specific standards are maintained throughout the screening programme, which must have a continuous programme quality assurance.

Different countries approach screening in different ways. Screening for a variety of different diseases has been established throughout India, including cancer, antenatal and newborn, child health, sexually transmitted diseases, and also a national screening programme for diabetic retinopathy.

Principles of screening. A WHO working paper published in 1968 considered various aspects of screening and determined a number of principles that will always be relevant to any screening programme in any health environment. However, as with many such principles, they cannot be universally applied to all situations, and exceptions occur, as will be seen in what follows. After taking into account international work on the appraisal of screening programmes, the NSC has added to the original principles. The principles concern the condition itself, the screening test, the treatment, and the screening programme.

UK NSC (NATIONAL SCREENING COMMITTEE) PRINCIPLES FOR SCREENING

The Condition

- The condition should be an important public health problem.
- The epidemiology and natural history of the condition, including development from latent to declared disease, should be adequately understood, and there should be a detectable risk factor, disease marker, latent period, or early symptomatic stage.
- All the cost-effective primary prevention interventions should have been implemented as far as possible.
- If the carriers of a mutation are identified as a result of screening, the natural history of people with this status should be understood, including any psychological implications.

The Test

- There should be a simple, safe, precise, reliable, robust, and validated screening test.

- The distribution of test values in the target population should be known, and a suitable cut-off level defined and agreed.
- The test should be acceptable to the population.
- There should be an agreed policy on the further diagnostic investigation of individuals with a positive test result and on the choices available to them.
- If the test is for mutations, but all possible known mutations are not being tested, the criteria used to select the subset of mutations to be covered by screening should be clearly set out.

The Treatment

- There should be an effective treatment or intervention for patients identified through early detection, with evidence of early treatment leading to better outcomes than late treatment.
- There should be agreed evidence-based policies covering which individuals should be offered treatment and the appropriate treatment to be offered.
- Clinical management of the condition and patient outcomes should be optimized in all healthcare providers prior to participation in a screening programme.

The Screening Programme

- There should be evidence from high-quality RCTs that the screening programme is effective in reducing mortality or morbidity. Where screening is aimed solely at providing information to allow the person being screened to make an "informed choice" (e.g. Down's syndrome, cystic fibrosis carrier screening), there must be evidence from high-quality trials that the test accurately measures risk. The information that is provided about the test and its outcome must be of value and readily understood by the individual being screened.
- There should be evidence that the complete screening programme (test, diagnostic procedures, treatment/intervention) is clinically, socially, and ethically acceptable to health professionals and the public.
- The benefit from the screening programme should outweigh the physical and psychological harm (caused by the test, diagnostic procedures, and treatment).
- The opportunity cost of the screening programme (include testing, diagnosis, and treatment, administration, training, and quality assurance) should be economically balanced in relation to expenditure on medical care as a whole (i.e. value for money). Assessment against these criteria should have regard to evidence from cost–benefit and/or cost-effectiveness analyses and have regard to the effective use of available resources.
- All other options for managing the condition should have been considered (e.g. improving treatment, providing other services) to ensure that no more cost-effective intervention could be introduced or current interventions increased within the resources available.

- There should be a plan for managing and monitoring the screening programme and an agreed set of quality assurance standards.
- Adequate staffing and facilities for testing, diagnosis, treatment, and programme management should be available prior to the commencement of the screening programme.
- Evidence-based information, explaining the consequences of testing, investigation, and treatment, should be available to potential participants to assist them in making an informed choice.
- Public pressure for widening the eligibility criteria for reducing the screening interval and for increasing the sensitivity of the testing process should be anticipated. Decisions about these parameters should be scientifically justifiable to the public.

The principles are specific to the UK but are relevant to most screening programmes in other countries. However, differing historical backgrounds to the ethical debate in other countries may result in different decisions about the implementation and application of screening.

2.12 CHANCE, BIAS, AND CONFOUNDING

Bias is the distortion of the estimated prevalence away from the true population value. It may arise because of how subjects are selected into the survey, and this is called selection bias. Alternatively, bias may arise as a result of how information is collected from the subjects, and this is called information bias.

Chance error. As mentioned, in most cross-sectional studies, a sample is drawn from the population and examined in detail; this is used to make inferences about the prevalence of disease in the general population. One of the most important concerns in any sampling procedure is therefore the avoidance of bias in selecting the sample so that it is reasonable to extrapolate results to the general population. The easiest and most acceptable way of avoiding such bias is for the sample to be drawn "at random," using a probability sampling scheme, which gives all eligible members of the population an equal or known probability of being selected. Given that a sample of n is drawn from a population of N individuals, the value p obtained from the sample (i.e. proportion with a disease) is considered as an estimate of the corresponding true value (P) in the population, with the expectation that some error may have occurred simply because of sampling variation. This type of error, known as sampling error (or random sampling error), arises entirely because only n members are measured instead of all N members. It is expected to occur because of chance differences between the members of the sample (n) and those not included in the sample. If all individuals in the population (N) were examined, there would be no sampling and no sampling error. When a probability sampling scheme has been used, the sampling error can be quantified and is usually presented in the form of "95% confidence limits" (95% CI) for the estimateed value; for example, the prevalence of blindness in population aged 50+ in India was estimated as 1.99%, with 95% CI of 1.94–2.13%. This indicates a probability of 0.95 that the reported limits contain the true population prevalence. Sampling error is thus a measure of precision because, other things being equal, the smaller it is, the closer the confidence limits and the more precise the estimate.

2.13 SOURCES OF BIAS

As mentioned earlier, non-sampling errors are difficult to quantify and may invalidate the survey findings. The main sources of such systematic errors in sample surveys are summarized here.

Selection bias. Biased selection of the eligible members of the population can be avoided by strict adherence to a well-devised random sampling scheme. The importance of allocating the predefined probability of selection to each sampling unit has been discussed earlier.

1. *Faulty coverage.* The term "under-coverage" refers to a situation where some of the eligible members of the population (eligible sampling units) are not included in the sampling frame and therefore are not given a chance to be selected. "Over-coverage" indicates the reverse, whereby members that are not eligible, for example, those outside the defined population, are included in the sampling frame (e.g. if people seeking eye care approach the survey team and are included in the sample). The problem, therefore, relates to the aptness of the sampling frame. The precise definition of the eligible members of the population (in terms of residence or other characteristics such as age) is a prerequisite.
2. *Non-response.* Many of the reports from the eye surveys mentioned earlier indicate that when a selected member cannot be "examined" because of absence or refusal or another difficulty, then every reasonable effort (with due regard to resources and to the ethics of the situation) is first made to enable an examination to take place. Substituting the next-door neighbour or arbitrary selection of another member may cause bias. If necessary, an additional eligible member may be selected randomly from the sampling frame; however, this is not a substitute for efforts to maximize response, since people who respond may be different from those who do not respond in terms of prevalence and risk factors for blindness, which could result in bias. Many of the recent eye surveys in developing countries have managed to minimize the non-response, having examined more than 90% of all those who were selected. By contrast, some eye surveys in urban settings, particularly in large metropolitan areas, have examined only about 60% of the selected sample. Surveys that involve house-to-house visits by the team tend to achieve a better response rate. When persons are invited to attend examination in a remote centre, or when postal questionnaires are used, the response generally tends to be poorer. In the well-designed eye survey RAAB study in India, 93,018 individuals ($\geq$50 years of age) were enumerated from 31 districts, out of which 85,135 completed all study procedures and ophthalmic assessment (participation rate 91.5%). This study has relied on media publicity and public relations to help provide information to the community and to secure the cooperation of community leaders and other key officials.

3. *Other sources of bias.* Other sources of information bias include systematic mistakes in measurement, diagnosis, and the classification of individuals, mistakes in recording data, and mistakes in data analysis and reporting. These errors could mean that the estimates of prevalence and causes of blindness from the survey do not reflect the true values in the total population. Procedures that may help estimate these sources of bias include:

- Preparation of a detailed protocol (manual of operations) for training and reference.
- Training of the members of the survey team in standardized methods of examination, grading, and classification, and assessing the level of agreement between the examiners (observers), before and during the survey, using observer agreement studies.
- Making the examinations and assessments as objective and as automated as possible. This may include (when possible) the use of image-capture systems (such as fundus camera) and subsequent "reading" of the images by an expert group, or a computerized image-analysis system.
- Data entry (manual or by scanning of the record sheet) using software with range checks and validity checks, and double data entry or formal checking of entered data against original records.

A glance at the studies described earlier will show that many are not representative of the general population, but that districts and sub-districts are generally chosen for convenience or because of a particular interest. Results from the National Blindness Survey in India (2015–2019) demonstrate that major differences can exist between regions of the country (10). These variations could partly result from sampling variations, as well as from real differences in prevalence between areas. In extrapolating the results of a local survey to a whole country, assumptions are made that may not be valid without further information. Similarly, results from one country cannot always be extrapolated to a whole region.

The published surveys have tended to favour rural areas, to the exclusion of urban vulnerable population. This is partly because the burden of avoidable blindness in developing countries has been thought to be higher in rural than urban parts of the country. It is perhaps also because it is easier to carry out a census and to identify the participants in rural villages than in multi-storied apartment buildings in a town, and because the response rate is usually better.

Ascertainment of prevalence of blindness in children presents special problems. With an average prevalence of less than one blind person (0.5 per 1,000) aged 0–49 years in India (10), it is not possible to examine several thousand children to find just a single case of blindness. Some studies use the age structure of a country to extrapolate the measured prevalence to an all-age population. However, even with a good knowledge of the age structure of the population of the country, only an estimated figure can be given, since firm data are not available for blindness in the younger age group.

In practice, many population surveys do not include visual field testing because of the time and cost involved, so that VA alone is used when deciding who is blind.

Publication bias. Many surveys on blindness that have been conducted have not been published in scientific journals. There may be a variety of reason for this, but the consequence is that the methodology cannot be examined, and the results are not available for use in global comparison or in the effort to eliminate blindness.

Confounding factors. Most published reports of epidemiological studies include estimation of the risk ratio, rate ratio, or odds ratio after adjustment for other factors besides the exposure of interest that may influence the association (these are called confounders or third factors that could explain the association between the exposure and the disease). For example, the decreasing prevalence of blindness in India cannot be solely attributed to the control interventions. There might be improvements in the socioeconomic fabric of society owing to the adoption of a market economy and the subsequent steep increase in industrial growth in the country, as well as a sudden improvement in life expectancy. It therefore becomes difficult to attribute the success or failure of a control programme directly to the programme itself if other relevant changes are occurring at the same time (confounding factors).

Recall and observer bias. It is inevitable that there will be some inaccuracies in the information reported by respondents for some, if not all, of the exposures. This is not confined to case-control studies. The critical question is whether inaccuracies in the reporting of exposure are different between cases and control, known as recall bias. Cases, in particular, may be influenced in their answers by awareness of being a case. A question on family history of a disease may have more incorrect positive responses in cases than controls because cases are seeking an explanation of why they have the disease.

Errors can also be introduced by observers, for example, by incorrect recording of information or variation in how interviews are conducted. Similar to recall bias, observer bias occurs when observer error differs proportionately between cases and controls. For example, interventions may be more likely to stress the importance of accurate information to cases, but not to controls.

How do inaccuracies in measurement affect the odds ratio? If errors by respondents or observers are proportionately similar between cases and controls (known as non-differential measurement error), then in general, but not invariably, the odds ratio will be reduced towards null (1.0). If recall or observer bias has occurred (known as differential measurement error), the odds ratio will be biased upwards or downwards, dependent on the direction of the bias. Unfortunately, since we do not know if recall or observer bias has occurred, we will not know if the odds ratios are biased or not. Errors in the measurement of confounders attenuate the adjustment for the effects of the confounding, resulting in "residual confounding." This produces bias in either direction, depending on the direction of the confounding. Researchers try to minimize the possibility of biases and errors by tactics such as keeping interviewers, cases, and controls masked with respect to the study hypotheses and by careful attention to questionnaire design and wording and to standardization of methods if physical or biological data are being collected. Rigorous training and quality control of all concerned with the collection of study data is essential.

Lost to follow-up. LFU can be a problem in the interpretation of the results. If those who are lost are more likely (or less likely) to have developed the disease than those who remain in the cohort, then this could introduce bias in our estimate of incidence. For example, if those lost were more likely to develop the disease, then we would underestimate the incidence of disease in our cohort. Of even greater concern is when LFU is higher in the exposed group compared with the unexposed group. For these reasons, investigators make great efforts to maximize the follow-up of their cohort participants.

2.14 TESTS OF SIGNIFICANCE

Most data from well-designed and executed clinical trials require only simple statistical methods for the analysis of independent or paired (correlated) data. Methods for comparison of independent groups (χ^2 test of independence, t-test, Wilcoxon Rank Sum Test, logrank test) may be used for clinical trials involving only one eye per person and those involving a person-specific outcome measure (e.g. quality-of-life score). Methods for comparison of correlated groups (McNemar's test for paired proportions, paired t-test, Wilcoxon Signed Rank Test) may be used for trials involving treatment of one eye with one treatment and the contralateral eye with the alternative treatment. When both eyes of the patient are assigned the same treatment and the outcome measure may be assessed on each eye, either one person-specific score may be used (the average of two eyes, or worst eye, or composite score), or the score from each eye may be analyzed using methods that account for the correlation between eyes. The choice of approach should be tied to the exact objective of the trial and the formulation of the primary outcome measure. Fortunately, there have been many advances incorporated into the major statistical software packages to deal with the analysis of correlated data.

Recruitment of patients may take place over months or years so that patients have varying length of follow-up. Survival analysis methods, such as the Kaplan–Meier method and Cox proportional hazards regression, accommodate varying lengths of follow-up. The outcome measure must be specified as a binary event, and the methods are valid only on the assumption that the reason for the varying length of follow-up is not related to the outcome, so that missed visits and loss to follow-up are not to be related to whether the patient's status is good or bad. Recent advances in the analysis of repeated measures of data, continuous or categorical, also accommodate varying lengths of follow-up.

REFERENCES

1. Frérot M, Lefebvre A, Aho S, Callier P, Astruc K, Glélé SA. What is epidemiology? Changing definitions of epidemiology 1978–2017. PLoS One. 2018;13(12).
2. Park K. Park's Textbook of Preventive & Social Medicine. 23rd ed. Bhanot; 2015. 14 p.

3. Johnson GJ, Minassian DC, Weale RA, West SK. The Epidemiology of Eye Disease. 3rd ed. Imperial College Press; 2012.

4. Mactaggart I, Limburg H, Bastawrous A, Burton MJ, Kuper H. Rapid assessment of avoidable blindness: looking back, looking forward. Br J Ophthalmol. 2019;103(11):1549–52.

5. Gupta N, Vashist P, Malhotra S, Senjam SS, Amit Bhardwaj VM. Rapid assessment of visual impairment in urban population of Delhi, India. PLoS One. 2015;10(4):1–11.

6. Vashist P, Senjam SS, Gupta V, Gupta N, Kumar A. Definition of blindness under National Programme for Control of Blindness: do we need to revise it? Indian J Ophthalmol. 2017;65(2):92–6.

7. Abou-Gareeb I, Lewallen S, Bassett K, Courtright P. Gender and blindness: a meta-analysis of population-based prevalence surveys. Ophthalmic Epidemiol. 20011;8:39–56.

8. Runda N, Manna S, Vanathi M, Tandon R, Gupta N. Tear film lipid layer thickness measurement from Ocular Surface Analyzer as a marker to monitor treatment of meibomian gland dysfunction in a study comparing physiological detergent-free eyelid wipes with conventional therapy: a randomized trial. Indian J Ophthalmol. 2022;70:1963.

9. Sommer A, Tarwotjo I, Djunaedi E, West KPJ, Loeden AA, Tilden R, et al. Impact of vitamin A supplementation on childhood mortality. A randomised controlled community trial. Lancet (London, England). 1986;1(8491):1169–73.

10. Vashist P, Senjam SS, Gupta V, Gupta N, Shamanna BR, Wadhwani M, Shukla P, Manna S, Yadav S, Bharadwaj A. Blindness and visual impairment and their causes in India: results of a nationally representative survey. PLoS One. 2022;17(7):e0271736.

11. Saxena R, Vashist P, Tandon R, Pandey RM, Bhardawaj A, Gupta V, et al. Incidence and progression of myopia and associated factors in urban school children in Delhi: the North India Myopia Study (NIM Study). PLoS One. 2017;12(12):e0189774.

12. Gupta SK, Gupta SC, Agarwal R, Sushma S, Agrawal SS, Saxena R. A multicentric case-control study on the impact of air pollution on eyes in a metropolitan city of India. Indian J Occup Environ Med. 2007;11(1):37–40.

13. Vashist P, Tandon R, Murthy GVS, Barua CK, Deka D, Singh S, et al. Association of cataract and sun exposure in geographically diverse populations of India: the CASE study. First Report of the ICMR-EYE SEE Study Group. PLoS One. 2020;15(1):e0227868.

14. Podgor MJ, Leske MC, Ederer F. Incidence estimates for lens changes, macular changes, open-angle glaucoma and diabetic retinopathy. Am J Epidemiol. 1983;118(2):206–12.

15. Klein BEK, Klein R, Lee KE. Incidence of age-related cataract: the beaver dam eye study. Arch Ophthalmol. 1998;116:219–25.

16. Panchapakesan J, Mitchell P, Tumuluri K, Rochtchina E, Foran S, Cumming RG. Five year incidence of cataract surgery: the Blue Mountains Eye Study. Br J Ophthalmol. 2003;87(2):168–72.
17. Miettinen OS. Proportion of disease caused or prevented by a given exposure, trait or intervention. Am J Epidemiol. 1974;99(5):325–32.
18. NHS screening—NHS [Internet]. [cited 2022 Aug 1]. Available from: www.nhs.uk/conditions/nhs-screening/

3

Epidemiological Principles Applied to Eye Diseases: Blindness and Visual Impairment

NOOPUR GUPTA, SUMIT GROVER, MEENAKSHI
WADHWANI, NAWAZISH SHAIKH

With the adoption of the Sustainable Development Goals and the growing recognition that health systems must strive to provide every individual the highest possible level of healthy functioning around the world, there is a need to measure and classify visual impairment (VI) and other aspects of health in a uniform fashion across all populations. Universality of classification has also been recognized as a fundamental underlying principle in the International Classification of Functioning, Disability, and Health. Standardizing the measurement and classification of VI and blindness is essential for meaningful comparisons of the burden of blindness across countries and regions (1–3).

3.1 CATEGORIES OF VISUAL IMPAIRMENT, INCLUDING BLINDNESS

The definition of visual impairment and blindness according to ICD-10, and used by WHO and recently endorsed by the National Program for Control of Blindness (NPCB), is described in Table 3.1. This is based on presenting visual acuity (PVA) and has been divided into the following categories.

3.1.1 Blindness

Blindness is defined as presenting visual acuity (PVA) of less than 3/60 in the better eye with available correction and visual field of less than 10 degrees from the point of fixation.

DOI: 10.1201/9781003291626-3

Table 3.1 Categories of Visual Impairment and Blindness as per ICD-10 (4)

Category	Presenting Distance Visual Acuity	
	Worse Than	Equal to or Better Than Snellen's Equivalent (logMAR)
0 = Mild or no visual impairment		6/18 3/10 (0.3) 20/70
1 = Moderate visual impairment	6/18 3/10 (0.3) 20/70	6/60 1/10 (0.1) 20/200
2 = Severe visual impairment	6/60 1/10 (0.1) 20/200	3/60 1/20 (0.05) 20/400
3 = Blindness	3/60 1/20 (0.05) 20/400	1/60* 1/50 (0.02) 5/300 (20/1200)
4 = Blindness	1/60* 1/50 (0.02) 5/300 (20/1200)	Light perception
5 = Blindness	No light perception	
9	Undetermined or unspecified	

3.1.2 Visual Impairment

Visual impairment is defined as presenting visual acuity less than 6/18 in the better eye.

Early visual impairment (EVI) is defined as presenting visual acuity of less than 6/12–6/18 in the better eye with available correction.

3.1.3 WHO Functional Definition of Low Vision (FLV)

A person with impairment of visual functioning even after treatment and/or standard refractive correction and a pinhole visual acuity of less than 6/18 to light perception, or a visual field of less than 20 degrees from the point of fixation, but who uses, or is potentially able to use, vision for planning and/or execution of a task.

3.1.4 Types of Blindness

Blindness may also be classified conceptually into the following categories based on visual acuity and activity restriction and community participation goals.

Economic blindness. The level of blindness that prevents an individual from earning wages; vision less than 6/60, with best correction in the better eye. This is also called work vision.

Social blindness. Vision of 3/60 or diminution of field of vision to 10 degrees. It is also called walk vision.

Manifest blindness. The level of blindness due to the best corrected visual acuity of 1/60 in the better eye.

Absolute blindness. The level of blindness due to the absence of perception of light in the better eye.

Legal blindness. The level of blindness that necessitates welfare measures. Vision less than 6/60 in the better eye with best correction and visual field less than 10 degrees.

Irreversible/non-avoidable blindness. The blindness that cannot be treated or prevented despite maximal therapy, for example, congenital anophthalmos.

Curable blindness. The blindness that is reversible by prompt management, for example, cataract.

Preventable blindness. That stage of blindness that could have been completely prevented by effective preventive/prophylactic measures, for example, retinopathy of prematurity, vitamin A deficiency.

Avoidable blindness. The sum of preventable and curable blindness. In developing countries, 85– 95% of blindness is avoidable.

3.2 RISK FACTORS AND CAUSES

Older age, female gender, illiteracy, and rural residence contribute to higher prevalence of blindness. Causes of blindness may vary in different geographical locations. The major causes of blindness in various regions are listed in Table 3.2.

3.3 EPIDEMIOLOGICAL DATA COLLECTION ON THE MAGNITUDE OF BLINDNESS

The data can be collected in different ways:

1. *Registry.* There are few registries that maintain the amount of blindness of their countries, but this number is generally incomplete due to a lack of

Table 3.2 Geographical Distribution of Causes of Blindness

Area	Causes
Asia	Cataract, trachoma, corneal disease, glaucoma, and vitamin A deficiency
Africa	Cataract, trachoma, corneal disease, glaucoma, vitamin A deficiency, onchocerciasis
Latin America	Cataract, glaucoma, diabetic retinopathy
North America + Europe	ARMD, diabetic retinopathy glaucoma

personal information on type, visual acuity, and causes of blindness. They are a source of robust, long-term data.

2. *Hospital-based studies.* It is not advisable to depend on hospital-based statistics as it includes a biased population. It may provide a rough estimate of the disease burden in the region but may reflect severe cases of the disease and those who have access to the healthcare service facility.

3. *Population-based surveys.* As per WHO, a population-based survey is an ideal and reliable method to extrapolate the correct magnitude of blindness. Rapid assessment surveys like Rapid Assessment of Avoidable Blindness (RAAB), Rapid Assessment of Visual Impairment (RAVI), and Rapid Assessment of Avoidable Visual Impairment (RAAVI), are rapid, economical, and reliable methods of finding prevalence of blindness and VI (5).

3.4 EPIDEMIOLOGICAL PRINCIPLES APPLIED TO CATARACT

Cataract can significantly affect an individual's mobility as well as quality of life and hence remains an important public health problem. Increased life span has the inevitable side effect of increased prevalence of cataract. Following the global trend, cataract remains as the leading cause of blindness and visual impairment in India even though there is a cost-effective intervention to circumvent the disease. Risk factors for the development of cataract include age, ultraviolet exposure, smoking, and exposure to indoor kitchen smoke (6).

3.4.1 Prevalence

The recent National Blindness and Visual Impairment Survey in India 2015–2019 (NPCB&VI 2015–2019) (7) showed the prevalence of blindness in population aged ≥50 years was 1.99%, whereas that for general population was 0.36%. Cataract in one or both the eyes was responsible for 66.2% of blindness, with the prevalence of bilateral cataract blindness being 0.84% (7).

INDICATORS OF CATARACT BLINDNESS AND SERVICE DELIVERY

1. **Cataract Surgical Rate (CSR)**

$$\frac{\text{Total number of cataract surgeries performed}}{\text{Total population above 50 years}} \times 1,000,000$$

2. **Sight Restoration Rate**

$$\text{Persons blind preoperatively} - \text{persons blind post operatively} \times 100$$

3. Cataract Surgical Coverage (CSC)

Measures the number of people in a population who have been operated for cataract as a proportion to all people operated or still requiring surgery and calculated as follows:

$$CSC = \left[(x+y)/(x+y+z) \right] * 100\,(\%)$$

Where:

x = bilateral operated (pseudophakic/aphakic)
y = unilateral operated (pseudophakic/aphakic) and other eye has operable cataract
z = bilateral cataract

Drawbacks of CSC

- Ignores quality of surgery.
- Person may still be visually impaired despite surgery, due to co-morbidities, residual refractive error, and post-operative complications.

4. Effective Cataract Surgery Coverage (eCSC)

WHO has recently identified effective cataract surgery coverage (eCSC) as a global indicator for monitoring progress towards universal eye health. It is now possible from the data analysis of population-based surveys to calculate this indicator that combines CSC with a measure of surgical quality in the form of visual outcome. eCSC is defined as the proportion of adults aged 50 years and older who are in need of cataract surgery, who have received this surgery, and who have a resultant good-quality distance visual acuity outcome.

WHO targets for 30% increase in effective cataract surgery coverage for all countries by the year 2030.

$$eCSC = \left[(a+b)/(c+d+e) \right] * 100$$

Where:

a = individuals with unilateral operated cataract attaining PVA ≥6/12 in the operated eye, who have BCVA <6/12, with cataract as the main cause of vision impairment or blindness in the other eye
b = individuals with bilateral operated cataract attaining PVA ≥6/12 in at least one eye
c = individuals with unilateral operated cataract (regardless of visual acuity in the operated eye) who have BCVA <6/12, with cataract as the main cause of vision impairment or blindness in the other eye
d = individuals with bilateral operated cataract, regardless of visual acuity
e = individuals with BCVA <6/12, with cataract as the main cause of vision impairment or blindness in both eyes

3.4.2 Conclusion

Cataract blindness remains one of the most common causes of blindness around the world. Ultraviolet radiation protection has an important role in tropical countries like India (ICMR EYE SEE study), where exposure to UV radiation is higher (6). Cataract surgery is the only cost-effective solution to cataract blindness. With increase in the annual number of cataract surgeries, the outcome of cataract surgeries needs to be assessed, as complications such as corneal decompensation itself may contribute to blindness and visual impairment.

3.5 EPIDEMIOLOGICAL PRINCIPLES APPLIED TO REFRACTIVE ERRORS

Refractive error is the most common cause of visual impairment (vision < 6/18 in the better eye) around the world and also in India and South-East Asia region. Over a quarter of the outpatient attendance at all eye clinics and hospitals is due to refractive errors. The availability and access of infrastructure, services, trained manpower, cost of spectacles, and community awareness are an area of concern.

3.5.1 Prevalence

NPCB&VI (National Programme for Control of Blindness and Visual Impairment 2015–2019) national survey showed that of all the individuals examined, 11.5% had uncorrected refractive error and 74.2% had uncorrected presbyopia (7). A community-based visual impairment study conducted by Nirmalan et al. in South India reported refractive error as the major cause of visual impairment and ocular morbidity, respectively, in their study (8).

There are around 8 million children in the age group of 5 to 15 years that suffer from uncorrected visual acuity or inadequately corrected refractive error, with a global prevalence of 0.96%, with the highest prevalence reported in urban areas in South-East Asia and China. The number of people aged 16 to 39 years that are visually impaired due to refractive error is 1.1%. The prevalence of uncorrected refractive errors in the age group of 40 to 49 years is 2.45% (9).

In children aged 5 to 15 years, the prevalence of uncorrected refractive error leading to visual impairment is higher in urban areas as compared to rural areas. There could be increased prevalence of myopia in urban areas due to increased exposure to digital devices and near work required for education; in this age group, the prevalence of myopia reported in studies that used the same definitions and cut off levels ranges from 3% to 35 %, hypermetropia from 0.4% to 17%, astigmatism from 2.2% to 34%, depending on the region and urban/rural setting (9).

3.5.2 Monitoring Indicators for Refractive Error Coverage

Effective refractive error coverage (eREC) is a global indicator identified by WHO for monitoring progress towards universal eye health. WHO targets a 40% increase in eREC for all countries by the year 2030. *eREC* is defined as the proportion of people who have received refractive error services (i.e. spectacles, contact lenses, or surgery) and have a resultant good-quality outcome relative to the number of people in need of refractive error services.

$$eREC = \left[(a+b)/(a+b+c+d)\right]*100(\text{For distance})$$

Where:

a = individuals with UCVA <6/12 in the better eye who present with spectacles or contact lenses for distance and whose PVA ≥6/12 in the better eye (met need)
b = individuals with a history of refractive surgery whose UCVA is ≥6/12 in the better eye (met need)
c = individuals with UCVA <6/12 in the better eye who present with spectacles or contact lenses for distance or a history of refractive surgery and a PVA of <6/12 in the better eye but who improve to ≥6/12 on BCVA (undermet need)
d = individuals with UCVA <6/12 in the better eye who do not have distance correction but who improve to ≥6/12 on BCVA (unmet need)

3.6 EPIDEMIOLOGICAL PRINCIPLES APPLIED TO PRESBYOPIA

Presbyopia is an age-related public health concern which limits near vision tasks due to changes in the accommodative ability of the lens. Uncorrected presbyopia is the leading cause of visual impairment throughout the world. There are 1.8 billion people suffering from presbyopia globally as per global estimates (10). Presbyopia not only affects the quality of life of individuals but also takes a toll on the economy of the country as a whole, specifically low- and middle-income countries like India. Thus, addressing presbyopia is imperative for achieving the Sustainable Development Goals that strive for promoting health and well-being for all.

3.6.1 Monitoring Indicators for Presbyopia

Effective refractive error coverage (eREC) for near, defined as the proportion of adults who are in need of presbyopic spectacles, who have received spectacles, and who have a resultant good-quality near visual acuity, outcome is used to assess the coverage for presbyopia in adults aged 35 years and above.

$$eREC = \left[(a+b)/(a+b+c+d)\right]*100(\text{For near})$$

Where:

a = individuals with UCVA <N6 at 40 cms in the better eye who present with spectacles for near and whose PVA is ≥N6 in the better eye (met need)

b = individuals with distance BCVA of ≥6/12 in at least one eye who present with spectacles for near and whose PVA was <N6 in the better eye (undermet need)

c = individuals with distance BCVA of ≥6/12 in at least one eye who do not have correction for near and whose UCVA was <N6 in the better eye (unmet need)

3.6.2 Conclusion

Uncorrected refractive error remains one of the important causes of visual impairment in the world, with simple, cost-effective solution such as the use of glasses. The access and availability of infrastructure, along with trained manpower, is the need of the hour to combat this epidemic of refractive error.

3.7 EPIDEMIOLOGICAL PRINCIPLES APPLIED TO CORNEAL BLINDNESS

Blindness is a global public health concern that inordinately affects low- and middle-income countries. About 4.2% of global blindness, that is, 1.4 million blind people worldwide, suffer from corneal opacity (CO) and trachoma-related blindness (11). The complex etiopathogenesis and varied modes of presentation of corneal diseases make it difficult to determine the exact prevalence of corneal blindness and to categorize its severity (12). This is well illustrated by the higher prevalence of corneal blindness seen in rural populations, where access to proper healthcare is poor and under-reporting of diseases is the norm, especially in developing countries like India (13, 14).

3.7.1 Prevalence

Diseases affecting the cornea are a major cause of blindness worldwide, second only to cataract in overall importance (7). Unlike cataract blindness, the data on the prevalence of blindness due to corneal pathologies is limited. Population-based data from many regions of the world are lacking (Table 3.3). The estimated prevalence of corneal blindness is 0.3–1.3%, according to various population-based studies. A systematic review of 41 articles on childhood blindness between 1999 and 2012 found a strong variation in the anatomical site of blinding eye conditions among WHO world regions ranging from 28% of corneal causes for the African region to 3.9% for the European regions (15). Countries reporting the highest estimated corneal causes in this study were Ethiopia (62.4%), Myanmar (43.6%), Ghana (41.8%), Sudan (40.0%), North-East India (36.4%), and Nepal (35.8%) (15). A high prevalence of corneal blindness and moderate-severe visual impairment (0.38% [95% CI, 0.30–0.46]) was reported in a meta-analysis conducted in 22 countries of Asia, with the highest prevalence in India (0.88%; 95% CI, 0.38–1.57) and the lowest in Sri Lanka (0.05%; 95% CI, 0.00–0.11) (16).

Table 3.3 Population-Based Studies for Estimating Prevalence of Corneal
Blindness

Study	Region	Blindness (%)	Most Common Cause	Group Studied	Definition Used for Blindness	Age Group
1 Li et al. (2009) (17)	China	U/L, 0.16% B/L, 0.80%	Childhood microbial keratitis (39.6%)	Population-based	VA <3/60 in better eye	>50 years
2 Gupta et al. (2014) (18)	India	U/L, 0.45% B/L, 0.12%	Pseudophakic bullous keratopathy (46.2%)	Population-based	VA <3/60 in better eye	All ages
3 Wang et al. (2014) (14)	China	U/L, 0.2% B/L, 0.1%	Microbial keratitis (40%)	Population-based	VA <3/60 in better eye	All ages
4 Song et al. (19) (2014)	China	0.23% (in at least one eye)	Infectious corneal disease (36.4%)	Population-based	VA <3/60 in better eye	All ages
5 Sheng et al. (20) (2014)	China	U/L, 0.73% B/L, 0.02%	Infectious and immune corneal disease, trauma	Population-based	VA <3/60 in better eye	All ages
6 Seidu et al. (21) (2017)	Nigeria	1.1% (in at least one eye)	Microbial keratitis (36.4%)	Population-based	VA <3/60 in better eye	All ages

3.7.2 Etiological Factors

Recent population-based studies demonstrate that, currently, ocular trauma, infectious keratitis, bullous keratopathy, and corneal degenerations are responsible for the major burden of corneal blindness among the rural populations in developing countries (13, 22). In the Corneal Opacity Rural Epidemiological Study conducted in Northern India, Gupta et al. reported that the common causes of corneal opacity in a population study with 12,899 participants from rural India were: pterygium (34.5%), ocular trauma (22.3%), and infectious keratitis (14.9%) (13). Corneal diseases contributing to blindness were post-surgical bullous keratopathy (46.2%) and corneal degenerations (23.1%) (13). Other studies conducted in Southern India demonstrated that ocular trauma (59.5%) is the commonest cause of corneal blindness (23). Population studies in China report infectious keratitis to be the leading cause of corneal blindness (14, 24–28).

Trachoma, the most common infectious cause of blindness, has always been associated with female gender, poverty, poor sanitation, and low socioeconomic status (29–31). Environmental risk factors, including hygiene, sanitation, and access to water, are also important in influencing the transmission of the trachoma bacterium (32). With trachoma, an effective package of interventions is available, which prevents the transmission of infection through surgery, antibiotic administration (mass drug administration of azithromycin), facial cleanliness, and environmental sanitation interventions, such as availability of functional latrines and clean running water (the SAFE strategy). In sub-Saharan African countries, studies identified trachomatous corneal opacity as the leading cause of bilateral blindness and non-trachomatous corneal opacity as the leading cause of unilateral blindness among the corneal causes of blindness (33). Trachoma has been found to be the most important cause of corneal blindness in countries with poor access to healthcare facilities, such as the Pacific Islands, South-East Asia, and Tropical Latin America.

3.8 EYE BANKING

Corneal transplantation remains the mainstay treatment option for visual rehabilitation of patients with corneal blindness. Approximately 185,000 keratoplasty procedures are performed globally on an annual basis (34). However, it is interesting to note that on a global scale, only 1 in 70 of those who are cornea-blind actually receives the surgery (34). This realization comes from the fact that the majority of the burden is concentrated in countries with poor and rural economies, where access to technologically intensive eye banking system is sparse, despite the need for the same, being at its peak.

Quality donor corneal tissue is available for transplantation through an effective eye banking system. Eye banks are responsible for collecting, harvesting, and processing donor corneas and their further distribution to surgeons (35). A three-tier organizational structure is recommended for an efficient eye banking system which involves eye donation centres (EDC), eye banks (EB), and eye bank training centres (EBTC). A lack of awareness about corneal donation and corneal transplantation acts as a major barrier to eye donation. A study from India identified illiteracy and rural population as predictors of ignorance of eye donation (36).

The need of the hour is capacity building and training of corneal transplant surgeons, along with maintenance of registry of all individuals with corneal blindness, appropriate referral of cornea-blind individuals to corneal transplant centres, and establishing an effective network with primary-level centres and with health workers at the grassroot level, benefitting the farthest and most inaccessible regions, where burden of corneal blindness is the highest. Monitoring and quality assurance are an important building block of any eye banking system.

3.8.1 Conclusion

The key to curbing corneal blindness in developing countries is prevention. This represents an area of focused research to develop better and easily accessible preventive and therapeutic strategies that could help mitigate the burden of diseases, allowing alleviation of some load off the eye banking system. A better healthcare delivery network and primary healthcare services equipped with the means to effectively tackle treatable causes can prevent the development of corneal opacification and eventual blindness. Prevention of causative diseases seems to be the way to approach corneal blindness, especially in developing countries like India, where the huge demand for corneal transplantation largely shadows the slow development of technologically intensive eye banking services.

3.9 EPIDEMIOLOGICAL PRINCIPLES APPLIED TO GLAUCOMA

Glaucoma is a multifactorial, progressive eye condition with an end point leading to irreversible damage to the optic nerve. Without general awareness, regular eye examinations, and careful adherence to the management plan, vision can deteriorate progressively. In most cases, glaucoma is asymptomatic until the late stages of the disease, and diagnosis is frequently delayed, resulting in significant, irreparable damage to vision.

3.9.1 Definition and Classification

A clear definition is vital for epidemiological study of any eye disease. The estimated prevalence and incidence of any eye condition depend on the criteria used to define the disease. As a result of the difficulties experienced with determining the presence or absence of glaucoma in population-based prevalence surveys, many definitions were proposed, like the International Society for Geographic and Epidemiologic Ophthalmology (ISGEO) Congress in Amsterdam in 1998, where *glaucoma* was defined as an optic neuropathy characterized by specific structural findings in the optic disc and particular functional deficits in automated visual field testing. This concept of "end organ damage" provides a uniform definition across the different mechanisms by which glaucoma is caused. *Primary open-angle glaucoma* (POAG) is currently defined by the European Glaucoma Society as a chronic progressive optic neuropathy with characteristic morphological changes at the optic nerve head and retinal nerve fibre layer, in the absence of other ocular disease or congenital anomalies. Progressive retinal ganglion cell death and VF loss are associated with these changes (37).

Glaucoma was formerly regarded solely as the result of an abnormally high intraocular pressure (IOP). A number of prevalence surveys showed that, in some populations, the majority of those with open-angle glaucoma have IOP that is typically within the normal range (< mean IOP ± 2 SDs) (38). These observations have influenced the development of theories on the aetiology of glaucomatous optic neuropathy and have removed the artificial dichotomy inherent in past use of the term "normal tension glaucoma." Although IOP is an important risk factor for glaucoma, it should not be regarded as a defining characteristic of the disease.

Similar to its definitions, there exist many approaches to the classification of glaucoma (39). The most widely used classifications employ the concept of primary and secondary disease. "Primary" implies unknown aetiology, whereas "secondary" denotes glaucoma developing as a consequence of another, recognizable ocular or systemic disease. *Primary open-angle glaucoma* (POAG) is defined as optic nerve damage, increased IOP, and characteristic visual field defects in an eye which does not have evidence of angle closure on gonioscopy and where there is no identifiable secondary cause. *Primary angle-closure glaucoma* (PACG) is defined as optic nerve damage, increased IOP, and characteristic visual field defects in an eye with narrow anterior chamber angle, with appositional contact between the peripheral iris and posterior trabecular meshwork.

3.10 EPIDEMIOLOGY

For glaucoma, the 1984 estimate of 3 million blind was revised in 1990 to 5.2 million. Independently, Quigley analyzed the available data for glaucoma and projected a figure of 6.7 million blind from glaucoma by the year 2000 (40). Quigley recently estimated that there would be 60.5 million people with glaucoma in 2010, and 79.6 million by 2020, among whom 74% would have open-angle glaucoma (41). Confrontational testing was regarded as the only practical method under field conditions. Now that there is more interest in the prevalence of different types of glaucoma and portable perimeters are available, routine visual field testing is regarded as essential in a survey if the true prevalence of glaucoma and of glaucoma blindness is to be estimated. Just like for blindness, it appears that women carry a larger burden of glaucoma blindness due to longevity and disadvantages in socioeconomic/health beliefs (42, 43). Mongolia (Central Asian region) and Barbados (Caribbean region) are unusual among all the countries in that glaucoma accounts for 28–35% of blindness, the same as for cataract (44). Most of these cases are of angle-closure glaucoma in Mongolia, but open-angle glaucoma in Barbados (45). There was a striking contrast in the proportion of blindness attributable to glaucoma in two studies in Singapore. Among the Chinese, 60% of all blindness was due to glaucoma (95), while among the Malays, glaucoma was responsible for only 5% of blindness (46, 47). It is possible, however, that there could have been confounding factors, as the studies were conducted six years apart and the numbers of blind individuals were low.

In 2010, a meta-analysis reported that 2.1 million (95% CI: 1.9–2.6) people were blind, and 4.2 (95% CI:3.7,5.8) million were visually impaired due to glaucoma. Glaucoma caused worldwide 6.6% (95% UI:5.9,7.9) of all blindness in 2010, and 2.2% (95% CI: 2.0–2.8) of all moderate and severe visual impairment (MSVI). These figures were lower in regions with younger populations (<5% in South Asia) than in high-income regions with relatively old populations (>10%). From 1990 to 2010, the number of blind or visually impaired due to glaucoma increased by 0.8 million (95% CI: 0.7, 1.1), or 62%, and by 2.3 million (95% CI: 2.1, 3.5), or 83%, respectively. The percentage of global blindness caused by glaucoma increased between 1990 and 2010 from 4.4% (4.0, 5.1) to 6.6%. Age-standardized prevalence of glaucoma-related blindness and MSVI did not differ markedly between world regions or between women (48). The National Blindness Survey in India in 31 districts had reported that glaucoma causes 5.5% of blindness, 0.8% of MSVI, and 1.4% of VI (7).

3.11 SCREENING FOR GLAUCOMA

In 1968, Wilson and Jungner published 10 "principles" for evaluating screening programs, criteria widely used since then as the dictum for guiding population-based screening for the diseases (49). They concluded that continuous screening is not feasible for diseases like glaucoma, and opportunistic comprehensive eye examination is the most cost-effective strategy for the same.

3.11.1 Challenges and Way Forward

Since many cases of glaucoma go unidentified and untreated, attempts have been made to create effective screenings for glaucoma. Even in developed countries, it is estimated that 50% of glaucoma sufferers remain undetected (50). In addition to having low specificity and sensitivity, glaucoma screenings are problematic because they may unintentionally hinder people from seeking comprehensive eye exams. Therefore, rather than implementing glaucoma screenings, which have been identified by research studies to be ineffective, it is instead important to promote regular eye exams by ophthalmologists as part of opportunistic screening in adults. In addition to providing the illusion that a comprehensive eye exam may not be needed, glaucoma screenings are also ineffective because of the lack of follow-up that occurs after glaucoma signs are detected.

Advocacy and policy guidelines have to be framed by stakeholders to effectively implement awareness campaigns to combat this silent thief of vision. Looking forward, the involvement of non-ophthalmologist human resource can be vital in this regard. A well-trained optometrist can pick up symptoms of frequent changes in near glasses and unexplained headaches by a complete and concise history-taking. Adding tonometry and evaluation of disc and angle as a routine protocol of vision assessment and refraction helps in detecting many such underlying cases. Awareness campaigns play a key role in encouraging regular eye checks and creating felt need for eye examinations. Since screening of glaucoma in the community has many scientific and feasibility constraints, the primary comprehensive eye and vision examinations may be the most cost-effective way to detect glaucoma in a high-risk population.

3.12 EPIDEMIOLOGICAL PRINCIPLES APPLIED TO DIABETIC RETINOPATHY

Diabetic retinopathy (DR) is one of the most common microvascular complications associated with diabetes mellitus. DR is one of the leading causes of ocular morbidity leading to devastating burden on health infrastructure. India is emerging as the diabetic capital of the world.

3.12.1 Prevalence

The estimated prevalence of diabetes worldwide in 2019 was 463 million, which is projected to increase to 700 million in 2045 (51). Approximately, 34.6% of persons with diabetes will develop any type of diabetic retinopathy; 10.2% will develop vision-threatening diabetic retinopathy. According to Sankara Nethralaya Diabetic Retinopathy Epidemiology and Molecular Genetics Study (SN DREAMS II), the four years' incidence of diabetic retinopathy and cystoid macular oedema is 9.2% and 2.6%, respectively (52). According to the National Diabetic Retinopathy Survey of India 2015–2019, among population aged ≥50 years, the prevalence of diabetic retinopathy among diabetics was found to be 16.9%, with prevalence of sight-threatening DR at 3.6% (7).

The prevalence of diabetic retinopathy in India according to difference studies is shown in Table 3.4.

3.13 RISK FACTORS AND SOCIODEMOGRAPHIC DETERMINANTS

The occurrence of diabetic retinopathy is related to the duration of diabetics along with level of control of this disease. The relationship among blood pressure, blood lipids, and body mass index (BMI) is inconsistent. Besides this, advanced age, male gender, insulin treatment deranged testing and postprandial blood glucose, increased glycosylated haemoglobin, deranged total cholesterol, triglyceride, and systolic blood pressure are also predisposing factors for the development of diabetic retinopathy (58).

3.13.1 Conclusion

The burden of DM and DR in India as well as globally is substantial, which highlights the need to adopt a multisectoral and coordinated approach to reduce their prevalence. Early identification of diabetes mellitus and routine screening for DR, as well as availability of infrastructure and trained persons to treat advanced cases of DR, is of utmost importance.

3.14 EPIDEMIOLOGICAL PRINCIPLES APPLIED TO AGE-RELATED MACULAR DEGENERATION (ARMD)

Age-related macular degeneration (AMD) is the leading cause of vision loss in those aged 60 years or older, and the prevalence is expected to rise with the increase in life expectancy. India has about 77 million people at or above the age of 60 years, representing a large group vulnerable to vision-related disorders, and the number is estimated to reach 180 million by 2026. As reported

Table 3.4 Prevalence of Diabetic Retinopathy in India

Author (Year)	Objective	Subjects (Prevalence %)
Rema et al. (2000) (53)	To assess the prevalence of retinopathy in newly diagnosed South Indian type-2 diabetic patients attending a diabetic centre	448 (7.3)
Narendran et al. (2002) (54)	To estimate the prevalence of diabetic retinopathy among self-reported diabetics in a population of southern India	54,508 (26.2)
Rema et al. (2005) (55)	To assess the prevalence of diabetic retinopathy in type-2 diabetic subjects in urban India using four-field stereo colour	1,382 (17.6)
Raman et al. (2009) (52)	To estimate the prevalence of diabetic retinopathy in an urban Indian population older than 40 years	599 (18)
Wadhwani et al. (2016) (56)	To develop and implement a community-based programme for screening of diabetic retinopathy in urban populations of Delhi	9,435 (13.5)
Vashist et al. (2019) (57)	National Diabetic Retinopathy Survey among population aged ≥50 years	5,986/1,010 (16.9)

in population-based studies, the prevalence of AMD in India ranges from 39.5% to 0.3% (59). These proportions are likely to increase further with an increase in the proportion of aging populations. In epidemiological studies, AMD is usually graded according to the International AMD Epidemiological Study Group.

3.15 EPIDEMIOLOGICAL PRINCIPLES APPLIED TO CHILDHOOD BLINDNESS

Childhood blindness and visual impairment (VI) constitute a continuum that includes children with blindness and decreased visual acuity. Globally, 1.4 million children suffer from blindness, and it is estimated that almost two-thirds of these inhabit developing countries. As per WHO estimates, there are around 1.4 million blind and 17.52 million children suffering from moderate or severe visual impairment globally. In low-income countries with high "under 5" mortality rates, the prevalence is reported to be as high as 1.5 per 1,000 children, while in high-income countries, the prevalence is reported to be 0.3 per 1,000 (60–63).

3.16 PREVALENCE AND ETIOLOGICAL FACTORS

As the prevalence of blindness in children is much lower than that in adults, a larger sample size of children is required to provide accurate data on prevalence and causes of childhood blindness. Hence, population-based surveys on childhood blindness are few. Registration data of blindness and severe visual impairment of children in European countries suggests a prevalence of approximately 0.3 per 1,000 children. Data from studies in Nepal and Bangladesh have indicated that the prevalence of childhood blindness ranges between 0.6 and 1.1 per 1,000 children (62, 64).

The Indian perspective on childhood blindness and visual impairment is shown in Table 3.5. The current prevalence of blindness in children is estimated to be around 0.8/1,000 (61, 65, 66).

The causes of childhood blindness can also be classified as shown in Table 3.6.

A systematic review of published Indian surveys reporting prevalence and causes of childhood blindness revealed that the causes of childhood blindness have changed with improvement in socio-developmental indicators. Corneal causes contributing to the maximum burden of blindness in children have shifted to globe abnormalities, like anophthalmos and microphthalmos. This is encouraging, as the avoidable causes are reducing and irreversible causes of blindness, like retinal dystrophies, globe abnormalities, continue to rise. Uncorrected refractive error and retinopathy of prematurity are two avoidable causes of blindness and visual impairment in children which need urgent attention (71).

3.17 RETINOPATHY OF PREMATURITY (ROP)

Retinopathy of prematurity (ROP) is one of the leading causes of preventable blindness in children worldwide (72). Middle-income nations are currently experiencing epidemic levels of ROP, because greater access to neonatal intensive care units has improved survival rates of premature infants, but without systematic oxygen management protocols.

High-income nations are currently undergoing a "second epidemic" of ROP, where infants are even smaller and younger due to further advances in neonatology to allow micro-preemies to survive. The current ROP epidemic in middle-income nations is known as the "third epidemic." As an extension of this third epidemic, lower-income nations, where neonatal care has improved greatly, are starting to experience a new wave of ROP.

Table 3.5 Indian Perspectives on Childhood Blindness

Author, Year	Number of Examined Participants (Age Group)	Blindness Prevalence	Visual Impairment Prevalence
Murthy, 2002 (67)	1,13,514 (5–15)	2.2/1,000 (PVA <20/200 in better eye)	13.6/1,000 (PVA <=20/60 in better eye)
Dandona, 2002 (68)	3,994 (7–15)	2/1,000 (PVA <20/200 in better eye)	7.3/1,000 (PVA <=20/60 in better eye)
Nirmalan, 2003 (8)	9,035 (≤15)	0.62/1,000 (BCVA <20/400 in better eye)	2.05/1,000 (BCVA <=20/60 in better eye)
Dorairaj, 2008 (69)	8,684 (≤ 15)	1.06/1,000 (BCVA <20/400 in better eye)	3.34/1,000 (BCVA <=20/60 in better eye)
Kemannu, 2016 (70)	23,087 (≤15)	0.8/1,000 (BCVA <20/400 in better eye)	—

Table 3.6 Avoidable Causes of Childhood Blindness

Preventable

Corneal scarring due to:

- Vitamin A deficiency
- Measles
- Ophthalmia neonatorum
- Traditional practices
- Infective corneal ulcers

Intrauterine

- Rubella
- Toxoplasma
- Other teratogens (alcohol)

Perinatal

- ROP
- Birth hypoxia

Hereditary diseases (consanguineous/genetic)

Treatable

- Cataract
- ROP
- Uveitis
- Glaucoma
- Corneal diseases (corneal ulcers and opacity)

Retinopathy of prematurity (ROP) is a proliferative retinal vascular disease affecting the retina of preterm infants. The clinical spectrum of ROP varies from spontaneous regression to bilateral retinal detachment and total blindness. Between these two extremes lies the form of ROP, which is amenable to effective prevention control strategies and treatment.

India is home to the largest number of preterm births and neonates at risk of developing ROP; studies suggest that of all the 14.8 million preterm births globally, approximately 23.4% babies are born annually in India (73). The main causes for increased ROP burden are high rate of prematurity, with improved survival and lack of uniform ROP screening protocols.

ROP management stands as a good example of all the strategies for prevention; for example, it includes a smaller number of preterm births by good obstetric care—primary prevention, lesser number of ROP by excellent neonatal care, primary prevention. Screening and prompt referral for treatment—secondary prevention and vitreoretinal surgery and rehabilitation—constitute tertiary prevention.

3.17.1 Integration of ROP Services within Existing Health System

The MoHI&FW (Ministry of Health and Family Welfare, India), under the National Health Mission, launched the Rastriya Bal Swasthya Karyakram (RBSK) (National Integrated Child Health Program), an innovative and ambitious initiative which envisages child health screening and early intervention services, a systemic approach of early identification and link to care, support, and treatment. RBSK covers early detection and management of 4 Ds—defects at birth, diseases of childhood, deficiencies, and developmental delays—covering 29 conditions, including ROP. Under RBSK, follow-up of all registered children up to the age of seven years is essential to ensure healthy childhood development.

3.17.2 Conclusion

Blindness and refractive error among children are an important public health concern as they have deep impact on psychological, emotional, and socioeconomic growth to the family. Despite the various difficulties in tackling childhood blindness, it is imperative to provide holistic socioeconomic development through utilization of the various public health programs for child health as well as comprehensive eye care to bring about a lasting change in the prevalence of childhood blindness.

REFERENCES

1. Wadhwani M, Vashist P, Senjam SS, Gupta V, Saxena R, Tandon R. A population-based study on the prevalence and causes of childhood blindness and visual impairment in North India. Indian J Ophthalmol. 2021 Jun;69(6):1381–7.

2. Nirmalan PK, Thulasiraj RD, Maneksha V, Rahmathullah R, Ramakrishnan R, Padmavathi A, et al. A population based eye survey of older adults in Tirunelveli district of south India: blindness, cataract surgery, and visual outcomes. Br J Ophthalmol. 2002 May;86(5):505–12.

3. Dandona L, Dandona R, John RK. Estimation of blindness in India from 2000 through 2020: implications for the blindness control policy. Natl Med J India. 2001 Nov 1;14(6):327–34.

4. List of Official ICD-10 updates [Internet]. [cited 2023 Mar 2]. Available from: www.who.int/standards/classifications/classification-of-diseases/list-of-official-icd-10-updates

5. Wong TY, Hyman L. Population-based studies in ophthalmology. Am J Ophthalmol. 2008 Nov;146(5):656–63.

6. Association of cataract and sun exposure in geographically diverse populations of India: the CASE study. First report of the ICMR-EYE SEE Study Group—PMC [Internet]. [cited 2023 Mar 4]. Available from: www.ncbi.nlm.nih.gov/pmc/articles/PMC6977762/

7. Vashist P, Senjam SS, Gupta V, Gupta N, Shamanna BR, Wadhwani M, et al. Blindness and visual impairment and their causes in India: results of a nationally representative survey. PLoS One. 2022 Jul 21;17(7):e0271736.

8. Nirmalan PK, Vijayalakshmi P, Sheeladevi S, Kothari MB, Sundaresan K, Rahmathullah L. The Kariapatti Pediatric Eye Evaluation Project: baseline ophthalmic data of children aged 15 years or younger in Southern India. Am J Ophthalmol. 2003 Oct 1;136(4):703–9.

9. Global magnitude of visual impairment caused by uncorrected refractive errors in 2004—PubMed [Internet]. [cited 2023 Mar 2]. Available from: https://pubmed.ncbi.nlm.nih.gov/18235892/

10. Fricke TR, Tahhan N, Resnikoff S, Papas E, Burnett A, Ho SM, et al. Global prevalence of presbyopia and vision impairment from uncorrected presbyopia: systematic review, meta-analysis, and modelling. Ophthalmology. 2018 Oct;125(10):1492–9.

11. Flaxman SR, Bourne RRA, Resnikoff S, Ackland P, Braithwaite T, Cicinelli MV, et al. Global causes of blindness and distance vision impairment 1990–2020: a systematic review and meta-analysis. Lancet Glob Health. 2017 Dec;5(12):e1221–34.

12. Barbosa AP, Alves M, Furtado JMF, Adriano L, Nominato LF, Dias LC, et al. Corneal blindness in Plato's cave: the acting forces to prevent and revert corneal opacity. Part I: epidemiology and new physiopathological concepts. Arq Bras Oftalmol. 2020 Oct 8;83:437–46.

13. Gupta N, Vashist P, Tandon R, Gupta SK, Dwivedi S, Mani K. Prevalence of corneal diseases in the rural Indian population: the Corneal Opacity Rural Epidemiological (CORE) study. Br J Ophthalmol. 2015 Feb;99(2):147–52.

14. Wang H, Zhang Y, Li Z, Wang T, Liu P. Prevalence and causes of corneal blindness. Clin Experiment Ophthalmol. 2014 Apr;42(3):249–53.

15. Kong L, Fry M, Al-Samarraie M, Gilbert C, Steinkuller P. An update on progress and the changing epidemiology of causes of childhood blindness worldwide. J AAPOS Off Publ Am Assoc Pediatr Ophthalmol Strabismus Am Assoc Pediatr Ophthalmol Strabismus. 2012 Dec 1;16:501–7.

16. Tran TM, Duong H, Bonnet C, Kashanchi A, Buckshey A, Aldave AJ. Corneal blindness in Asia: a systematic review and meta-analysis to identify challenges and opportunities. Cornea. 2020 Sep;39(9):1196–205.

17. Li Z, Cui H, Zhang L, Liu P, Bai J. Prevalence of and associated factors for corneal blindness in a rural adult population (the southern Harbin eye study). Curr Eye Res. 2009 Aug;34(8):646–51.

18. Gupta N, Vashist P, Tandon R, Gupta SK, Dwivedi S, Mani K. Prevalence of corneal diseases in the rural Indian population: the Corneal Opacity Rural Epidemiological (CORE) study. Br J Ophthalmol. 2015 Feb;99(2):147–52.

19. Song X, Xie L, Tan X, Wang Z, Yang Y, Yuan Y, et al. A multi-center, cross-sectional study on the burden of infectious keratitis in China. PLoS One. 2014 Dec 1;9(12):e113843.

20. Sheng XL, Li HP, Liu QX, Rong WN, Du WZ, Ma L, et al. Prevalence and associated factors of corneal blindness in Ningxia in northwest China. Int J Ophthalmol. 2014 Jun 18;7(3):557–62.

21. Nigeria Seidu MA, Olusanya BA, Ogundipe AO. Prevalence and determinants of corneal blindness in a Semi-Urban population of southwest. Niger J Ophthalmol 2017;25:18–27. [Internet]. [cited 2023 Mar 4]. Available from: www.nigerianjournalofophthalmology.com/article.asp?issn=0189-9171;year=2017;volume=25;issue=1;spage=18;epage=27;aulast=Seidu

22. Mukhija R, Gupta N, Vashist P, Tandon R, Gupta SK. Population-based assessment of visual impairment and pattern of corneal disease: results from the CORE (Corneal Opacity Rural Epidemiological) study. Br J Ophthalmol. 2020 Jul;104(7):994–8.

23. Reddy TN, Anjaneyulu K, Vishnupriya S, Kanth CV, Nagarani K. Proportion of corneal blindness in blind patients attending for blind certificates in regional eye hospital, Kurnool. J Evol Med Dent Sci. 2017 Apr 13;6(30):2407–10.

24. Song X, Xie L, Tan X, Wang Z, Yang Y, Yuan Y, et al. A multi-center, cross-sectional study on the burden of infectious keratitis in China. PLoS One. 2014 Dec 1;9(12):e113843.

25. Cao J, Yang Y, Yang W, Wu R, Xiao X, Yuan J, et al. Prevalence of infectious keratitis in Central China. BMC Ophthalmol. 2014 Apr 2;14:43.

26. Li Z, Cui H, Zhang L, Liu P, Bai J. Prevalence of and associated factors for corneal blindness in a rural adult population (the southern Harbin eye study). Curr Eye Res. 2009 Aug;34(8):646–51.

27. Raj N, Gupta N, Kumar D, Vashist P, Tandon R. Population-based study on the prevalence, clinical characteristics and vision-related quality of life in patients with corneal opacity resulting from infectious keratitis: results from the Corneal Opacity Rural Epidemiological study. Br J Ophthalmol. 2021 Nov 12;107:476–82.

28. Sheng XL, Li HP, Liu QX, Rong WN, Du WZ, Ma L, et al. Prevalence and associated factors of corneal blindness in Ningxia in northwest China. Int J Ophthalmol. 2014;7(3):557–62.

29. Munoz B, Aron J, Turner V, West S. Incidence estimates of late stages of trachoma among women in a hyperendemic area of central Tanzania. Trop Med Int Health. 1997 Nov;2(11):1030–8.

30. Schwab L, Whitfield R, Ross-Degnan D, Steinkuller P, Swartwood J. The epidemiology of trachoma in rural Kenya. Variation in prevalence with lifestyle and environment. Study Survey Group. Ophthalmology. 1995 Mar;102(3):475–82.

31. Zerihun N. Trachoma in Jimma zone, south western Ethiopia. Trop Med Int Health. 1997 Dec;2(12):1115–21.

32. Stocks ME, Ogden S, Haddad D, Addiss DG, McGuire C, Freeman MC. Effect of water, sanitation, and hygiene on the prevention of trachoma: a systematic review and meta-analysis. PLoS Med. 2014 Feb;11(2):e1001605.

33. Porth JM, Deiotte E, Dunn M, Bashshur R. A review of the literature on the global epidemiology of corneal blindness. Cornea. 2019 Dec;38(12):1602–9.

34. Gain P, Jullienne R, He Z, Aldossary M, Acquart S, Cognasse F, et al. Global survey of corneal transplantation and eye banking. JAMA Ophthalmol. 2016 Feb;134(2):167–73.

35. Rao GN. What is eye banking? Indian J Ophthalmol. 1996 Mar;44(1):1–2.

36. Gupta N, Vashist P, Ganger A, Tandon R, Gupta SK. Eye donation and eye banking in India. Natl Med J India. 2018 Oct;31(5):283–6.

37. European Glaucoma Society terminology and guidelines for glaucoma, 4th Edition—Chapter 2: classification and terminology supported by the EGS Foundation. Br J Ophthalmol. 2017 May;101(5):73–127.

38. Comparison of glaucomatous progression between untreated patients with normal-tension glaucoma and patients with therapeutically reduced intraocular pressures. Collaborative Normal-Tension Glaucoma Study Group—PubMed [Internet]. [cited 2023 Mar 2]. Available from: https://pubmed.ncbi.nlm.nih.gov/9780093/

39. Foster PJ, Buhrmann R, Quigley HA, Johnson GJ. The definition and classification of glaucoma in prevalence surveys. Br J Ophthalmol. 2002 Feb;86(2):238–42.

40. Quigley HA. Number of people with glaucoma worldwide. Br J Ophthalmol. 1996 May;80(5):389–93.

41. Number of people with glaucoma worldwide—PubMed [Internet]. [cited 2023 Mar 2]. Available from: https://pubmed.ncbi.nlm.nih.gov/8695555/

42. Gender and blindness: a meta-analysis of population-based prevalence surveys—PubMed [Internet]. [cited 2023 Mar 2]. Available from: https://pubmed.ncbi.nlm.nih.gov/11262681/

43. Gender and glaucoma: what we know and what we need to know—PMC [Internet]. [cited 2023 Mar 2]. Available from: www.ncbi.nlm.nih.gov/pmc/articles/PMC4326058/

44. Glaucoma in Mongolia. A population-based survey in Hövsgöl province, northern Mongolia—PubMed [Internet]. [cited 2023 Mar 2]. Available from: https://pubmed.ncbi.nlm.nih.gov/8859083/
45. The Barbados Eye Study. Prevalence of open angle glaucoma—PubMed [Internet]. [cited 2023 Mar 2]. Available from: https://pubmed.ncbi.nlm.nih.gov/8002842/
46. Prevalence and causes of low vision and blindness in an urban malay population: the Singapore Malay Eye Study—PubMed [Internet]. [cited 2023 Mar 4]. Available from: https://pubmed.ncbi.nlm.nih.gov/18695104/
47. Causes of blindness, low vision, and questionnaire-assessed poor visual function in Singaporean Chinese adults: the Tanjong Pagar Survey—PubMed [Internet]. [cited 2023 Mar 2]. Available from: https://pubmed.ncbi.nlm.nih.gov/15177966/
48. Bourne RRA, Taylor HR, Flaxman SR, Keeffe J, Leasher J, Naidoo K, et al. Number of people blind or visually impaired by glaucoma worldwide and in world regions 1990–2010: a meta-analysis. PLoS One. 2016 Oct 20;11(10):e0162229.
49. Principles and practice of screening for disease [Internet]. [cited 2023 Mar 2]. Available from: https://apps.who.int/iris/handle/10665/37650
50. Health anxiety in a non-population-based, pre-publicised glaucoma screening exercise—PubMed [Internet]. [cited 2023 Mar 4]. Available from: https://pubmed.ncbi.nlm.nih.gov/19521429/
51. Saeedi P, Petersohn I, Salpea P, Malanda B, Karuranga S, Unwin N, et al. Global and regional diabetes prevalence estimates for 2019 and projections for 2030 and 2045: results from the International Diabetes Federation Diabetes Atlas, 9th ed. Diabetes Res Clin Pract. 2019 Nov;157:107843.
52. Raman R, Rani PK, Reddi Rachepalle S, Gnanamoorthy P, Uthra S, Kumaramanickavel G, et al. Prevalence of diabetic retinopathy in India: Sankara Nethralaya Diabetic Retinopathy Epidemiology and Molecular Genetics Study report 2. Ophthalmology. 2009 Feb;116(2):311–8.
53. Rema M, Deepa R, Mohan V. Prevalence of retinopathy at diagnosis among type 2 diabetic patients attending a diabetic centre in south India. Br J Ophthalmol. 2000 Sep;84(9):1058–60.
54. Narendran V, John RK, Raghuram A, Ravindran RD, Nirmalan PK, Thulasiraj RD. Diabetic retinopathy among self reported diabetics in southern India: a population based assessment. Br J Ophthalmol. 2002 Sep;86(9):1014–8.
55. Rema M, Premkumar S, Anitha B, Deepa R, Pradeepa R, Mohan V. Prevalence of diabetic retinopathy in urban India: the Chennai Urban Rural Epidemiology Study (CURES) eye study, I. Invest Ophthalmol Vis Sci. 2005 Jul;46(7):2328–33.
56. Wadhwani M, Vashist P, Singh SS, Gupta N, Malhotra S, Gupta A, et al. Diabetic retinopathy screening programme utilising non-mydriatic fundus imaging in slum populations of New Delhi, India. Trop Med Int Health. 2018 Apr;23(4):405–14.

57. Vashist P, Senjam SS, Gupta V, Manna S, Gupta N, Shamanna BR, et al. Prevalence of diabetic retinopahty in India: results from the National Survey 2015–19. Indian J Ophthalmol. 2021 Nov;69(11):3087–94.

58. Namperumalsamy P, Kim R, Vignesh TP, Nithya N, Royes J, Gijo T, et al. Prevalence and risk factors for diabetic retinopathy: a population-based assessment from Theni District, south India. Br J Ophthalmol. 2009 Apr;93(4):429–34.

59. Prevalence of early and late age-related macular degeneration in India: the INDEYE study—PubMed [Internet]. [cited 2023 Mar 4]. Available from: https://pubmed.ncbi.nlm.nih.gov/19696177/

60. Childhood blindness in the context of VISION 2020--the right to sight—PubMed [Internet]. [cited 2023 Mar 2]. Available from: https://pubmed.ncbi.nlm.nih.gov/11285667/

61. Visual impairment in childhood: insights from a community-based survey—PubMed [Internet]. [cited 2023 Mar 2]. Available from: https://pubmed.ncbi.nlm.nih.gov/14616907/

62. Visual impairment in children in middle- and lower-income countries—PubMed [Internet]. [cited 2023 Mar 2]. Available from: https://pubmed.ncbi.nlm.nih.gov/21868404/

63. Magnitude and temporal trends in Avoidable Blindness in Children (ABC) in India—PubMed [Internet]. [cited 2023 Mar 2]. Available from: https://pubmed.ncbi.nlm.nih.gov/28646264/

64. The key informant method: a novel means of ascertaining blind children in Bangladesh—PubMed [Internet]. [cited 2023 Mar 2]. Available from: https://pubmed.ncbi.nlm.nih.gov/17431019/

65. Causes and temporal trends of blindness and severe visual impairment in children in schools for the blind in North India—PMC [Internet]. [cited 2023 Mar 2]. Available from: www.ncbi.nlm.nih.gov/pmc/articles/PMC1771821/

66. A cross-sectional study of prevalence and etiology of childhood visual impairment in Auckland, New Zealand—PubMed [Internet]. [cited 2023 Mar 2]. Available from: https://pubmed.ncbi.nlm.nih.gov/26107975/

67. Murthy GVS, Gupta SK, Ellwein LB, Muñoz SR, Pokharel GP, Sanga L, et al. Refractive error in children in an urban population in New Delhi. Invest Ophthalmol Vis Sci. 2002 Mar;43(3):623–31.

68. Dandona R, Dandona L, Srinivas M, Sahare P, Narsaiah S, Muñoz SR, et al. Refractive error in children in a rural population in India. Invest Ophthalmol Vis Sci. 2002 Mar;43(3):615–22.

69. Childhood blindness in a rural population of southern India: prevalence and etiology—PubMed [Internet]. [cited 2023 Mar 4]. Available from: https://pubmed.ncbi.nlm.nih.gov/18569813/

70. Kemmanu V, Hegde K, Giliyar SK, Shetty BK, Kumaramanickavel G, McCarty CA. Prevalence of childhood blindness and ocular morbidity in a rural pediatric population in Southern India: the Pavagada Pediatric Eye Disease Study-1. Ophthalmic Epidemiol. 2016 Jun;23(3):185–92.

71. Wadhwani M, Vashist P, Singh SS, Gupta V, Gupta N, Saxena R. Prevalence and causes of childhood blindness in India: a systematic review. Indian J Ophthalmol. 2020 Feb;68(2):311.

72. Update on blindness due to retinopathy of prematurity globally and in India—PubMed [Internet]. [cited 2023 Mar 4]. Available from: https://pubmed.ncbi.nlm.nih.gov/27915313/

73. Retinopathy of prematurity: overview and highlights of an in . . . : Indian J Ophthalmol [Internet]. [cited 2023 Mar 4]. Available from: https://journals.lww.com/ijo/Fulltext/2021/02001/Retinopathy_of_prematurity__Overview_and.27.aspx

4

Epidemiological Research and Surveys in Eye Care

VIVEK GUPTA, SOUVIK MANNA, NOOPUR GUPTA,
PRAVEEN VASHIST

We have already discussed the uses of epidemiology, various study designs, and issues of bias in Chapter 2. In this chapter, we will focus on how to plan and conduct a research study.

4.1 BACKGROUND AND RESEARCH QUESTION

The idea for conducting a research may come from day-to-day clinical experiences, discussions with colleagues, reading other research papers, etc. Any well-planned research study proposal or paper will start by explaining the rationale or the need to conduct the study. This may include brief statements about the burden of that eye disease, current diagnostic/therapeutic choices, etc. (*what we know*). Then the gap in current knowledge is noted (*what we don't know*). Thus, the reasoning for conducting the study is conveyed.

Thereafter, it is helpful to state the research question. It is a clear articulation of the problem statement or the gap in the current knowledge that the research study aims to address. A question well asked is a question half-answered. The way the question (or hypothesis) is stated shows what data will be necessary to answer (or test) it and probably suggests also how and from where or from whom the data will be obtained. A good research question should be feasible, interesting, novel, ethical, and relevant (FINER). These points are elaborated in Table 4.1.

When writing a research question, the following should be included (PICO):

1. P: Who is the target population (e.g. persons with diabetes in the community, persons with diabetic retinopathy, schoolchildren, etc.)?

DOI: 10.1201/9781003291626-4

Table 4.1 Suggested Parameters to Consider while Developing a Research Question

Feasible	• Adequate number of study participants available willing to participate. • Do the investigator and colleagues have the skills and experience to design and carry out the study? • Affordable in time and cost; being realistic is important. • Has a testable hypothesis.
Interesting	• To the investigator. • To your peers/other researchers. • To the journal editors/reviewers. • To possible funders. • To policymakers.
Novel	• First ever study on this issue? • First ever study in your setting (which is very unique and has special characteristics by geography, populations served, etc.)? • Improving the methodology of previous studies to address previous limitations and obtain more valid findings?
Ethical	• A good research question MUST be ethical. • It must be able to be approved by your institutional review board (ethics committee). • Almost ALL research requires formal ethical review and a consent process.

Relevant	• Will your study findings:
	   • Influence practice guidelines?
	   • Influence health policy?
	   • Advance scientific knowledge?
	   • Guide future research?

2. I: What is the intervention or exposure (*will be missing in observational studies*, for example, strict control of blood sugar levels)?
3. C: The comparison: What is the comparison group (if applicable) (*will be missing in observational studies*, for example, uncontrolled blood sugar levels)?
4. O: What is the outcome or end point (prevalence of diabetic retinopathy, lower risk of sight-threatening diabetic retinopathy)?

Please read the following research questions and ask yourself what the PICO components within them are:

1. Does strict control of blood sugar lead to lower risk of sight-threatening diabetic retinopathy among persons with diabetic retinopathy when compared with uncontrolled blood sugar level?

2. What is the prevalence of uncorrected refractive error among school children in urban Delhi?
3. Is low education status a risk factor for delay in cataract surgery among elderly Indian population?

4.2 AIMS AND OBJECTIVES

A research aim expresses the overall intent or purpose of the study. It should be reasonably specific, and often, the research question, when expressed not as a question but as a statement, would be a good starting point. The aim describes the overarching goal of a research study.

After the aim come the objectives. Research objectives outline the specific steps that are needed to meet the research aim. If a research study has more than one objective, it is helpful to identify the most important one as the "primary objective" and the rest as "secondary objectives." As an example, some objectives of the National Survey of Blindness and Visual Impairment India were:

Primary Objectives

- To determine the prevalence of blindness and visual impairment among the 50-plus-year-aged population in India.
- To identify the major causes of blindness (including avoidable blindness) in India.

Secondary Objectives

- To assess the prevalence of diabetic retinopathy in the study population.
- To ascertain the visual outcomes after cataract surgery among operated cases.
- To estimate the cataract surgical coverage in different states of India.
- To identify the proportion of people with known diabetes who have had a previous fundus examination.

It is recommended that the objectives should be SMART: specific, measurable, achievable, realistic, and time-bound (Figure 4.1).

SMART Objectives

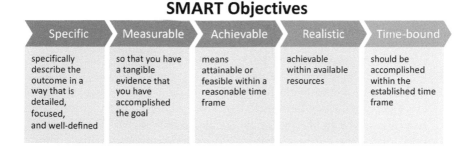

Specific	Measurable	Achievable	Realistic	Time-bound
specifically describe the outcome in a way that is detailed, focused, and well-defined	so that you have a tangible evidence that you have accomplished the goal	means attainable or feasible within a reasonable time frame	achievable within available resources	should be accomplished within the established time frame

Figure 4.1 Developing SMART objectives for a research study.

4.3 METHODS

Now that the objectives of the study are clear, one should develop a clear plan of how the study will be conducted. It is helpful to document the methods that will be followed under the following headings:

1. **Study design.** Whether it is cross sectional, case control, cohort, randomized controlled trial, etc.
2. **Study population.** The population to which the study results would be applicable.
3. **Study setting.** Describe where the study will be conducted. Is it a hospital, eye care centre, or a community-based setting (which part of the country, which state, etc.).
4. **Study variables.** List which are the variables of interest that will be measured or assessed in the study. Study variables include:
   a. *Outcome variables.* The main variable that we are interested in: prevalence of blindness, prevalence of myopia, quality of life, achieving target IOP, etc.
   b. *Exposure/intervention variables.* These are relevant only in case control, cohort, or experimental studies, for example, strict glycaemic control, parental myopia, outdoor activity, etc.
   c. *Risk factor (or explanatory) variables.* The variables that may affect are a risk factor for the outcome, OR, which may affect the relationship between the exposure and the outcome (potential confounder variables), for example, age, sex, education, socioeconomic status, smoking, etc.

For each variable, it is imperative that a clear definition for how it will be measured be decided upon and documented in the study plan. Example: DR will be diagnosed if any eye shows signs of mild NPDR or worse based on the ETDRS criteria.

5. **Study participants.** List what will be the inclusion and exclusion criteria based on which participants will be enrolled in the study. You may wish to include persons of certain age, gender, etc. and may wish to exclude persons with co-existing ocular conditions.
6. **Sample size calculation.** An estimation of how many participants you should include in the study to be able to derive statistically valid conclusions about the target study population.
7. **Sampling plan.** How the study participants will be enrolled in the study. In randomized controlled trial, describe how a participant will be allocated to either the intervention or the control treatment.
8. **Study tools.** These include the questionnaires that will be used, the ophthalmic clinical examinations, investigations, laboratory tests, etc. with exact steps that will be performed. For example, IND-VFQ questionnaire administered by an interviewer, monocular-presenting visual acuity using tumbling E chart at 6 m by trained field assistants, fasting capillary blood glucose using portable glucometer, objective retinoscopy using streak retinoscope at 50 cm by optometrist, etc. Documenting these is necessary to

remove ambiguity in the assessment methods and to ensure all participants get evaluated using similar techniques. You should also sample questionnaires as annexures to the study plan.

9. **Procedures.** In this section, prepare a step-by-step account of how the study will be done.
   a. Describe the composition of the study team who will collect data and perform clinical examinations.
   b. Describe how the staff will be trained, who will do the training, and the duration of the same.
   c. Pilot testing or pretesting. Often, in large studies, there is a testing of the study protocol before actual data collection for the main study is initiated. This helps in identifying and ironing out the issues in the study methodology.
   d. Step-by-step, the procedure to be followed right from participant identification, obtaining consent, sequence of administration of study tools and assessments, etc., right till completion of data collection from that patient. It is very useful to present the study methodology as a flow chart.
   e. Steps to ensure quality of data collected. Include a plan for supervision and monitoring of data collection, especially if the research team has multiple staff members. Document what you feel are any foreseeable barriers in carrying out the research study—for example, attrition in follow-up studies, refusals, persons in jobs and therefore not available at home. Then list out the steps that will be taken to minimize the impact of such barriers.

10. **Data entry and analysis.** Data entry in a research study can be done using Microsoft™ Excel or using special tools dedicated for research data entry. It is vital to ensure that correct data is entered and transcription errors be minimized. Appropriate statistical analysis needs to be done. When developing proposal, it is useful to develop a data analysis plan listing the incidence, prevalence, etc. calculations that will be done and statistical tests that will be used for comparisons. Many researchers even develop a template of tables of results that can guide the data analysis. Data analysis can be done using specialized software, such as R, Stata, etc.

11. **Ethics.** Globally, certain principles of research ethics have been recognized. Participants should be informed that they are being invited to join a research study, why that study is needed, and they should be free to decide whether they wish to enrol in the study on their own free will, without fear or repercussions. A written informed consent must be obtained. In addition, the researcher should also make provision for treatment of any research-related injuries.

4.4 SAMPLE SIZE

A sample size will depend upon the desired level of precision for estimating prevalence, the sampling scheme, the population size, and cost and logistic issues. Having devised an efficient sampling scheme (one that would result in minimal sampling error for any given sample size and cost), an approximate minimum sample size, required to give the desired precision, may be calculated using standard statistical tools which are widely available. The equations require the following criteria to be specified:

- The expected prevalence of the condition in the population. This is usually based on the results of surveys conducted in similar settings.
- The desired precision (the maximum sampling error that is acceptable) for estimating the prevalence of the disorder(s) deemed as "most appropriate" in the objective of the study. Calculations are also made for the secondary objectives. The desired precision will strongly depend upon the "expected" prevalence in the population: for example, when the prevalence is expected to be in the region of 0.1 (i.e. 10%), a sampling error of ±0.02 may be acceptable, whereas a much smaller sampling error (e.g. ±0.005) is required for an expected prevalence of, for example, 0.025. Calculations are usually made for several different assumed values of the prevalence and the corresponding levels of precision.
- The power of the study (i.e. the probability that the test will reject the null hypothesis when the alternative hypothesis is true), insofar as it relates to the probability of not exceeding the specified sampling error. This is usually fixed at 0.95 (for 95% confidence limits), in contrast to the flexibility in other types of study, such as clinical trial, or cross-sectional study for estimation of an effect measure.
- The population size, because larger sampling fractions (n/N) tend to yield smaller sampling errors. This may have a negligible effect on the sample size when N is very large.
- The expected design effect. It may be difficult to predict a value for this with any level of certainty, but instances of the actual findings in other similar studies may be useful. Unfortunately, very few eye surveys have reported the observed design effect.

A number of readily available statistical software packages, such as Open-Epi, may be used to compute sample size. The design effect (D_{eff}) is important in calculating the required sample size for a planned survey. If the anticipated D_{eff} is underestimated, or if no allowance is made for it, then the desired precision may not be attained, and the 95% CI for the prevalence estimate may be considerably wider than hoped for.

Design effect. The random sampling errors in CLS depend not only on the size of the clusters but also on the sum of the differences between the overall prevalence and the prevalence in each cluster. In general, when such differences are large and numerous, the random sampling error is also large. The design effect (D_{eff}) is a ratio of two variances (measure of random sampling error) V_1/V_2, where V_1 is the variance when a CLS method has been used, and V_2 is calculated assuming an SRS mwthod and gives a measure of how highly clustered a condition is within communities. The D_{eff} is close to 1.0 when a CLS method has been employed.

The following equation is intended to help the understanding of the relationship between sample size and its determinants (excluding any stratification).

$$n = \frac{t^2 PQW / E^2}{\left(1 + \dfrac{1}{N}\right)\left(\left(\dfrac{t^2 PQW}{E^2}\right) - 1\right)}$$

Where n is the minimum sample size required (approximate), P is the assumed prevalence in the population (a proportion), Q is $1-P$, E is the maximum random sampling error acceptable, W is the likely design effect, N is the population size, and t is the standardized normal deviate, usually fixed at 1.96, to give 95% probability of not exceeding E.

When N is very large in relation to n (e.g. N is more than a million and $n <$ 3,000), the denominator of the equation will have a value very close to 1.0, giving a simpler equation:

$$n = \frac{t^2 PQW}{E^2}$$

Alpha level is the probability of a type I error, that is, falsely rejecting the null hypothesis. Usually, we consider an alpha level of at least 0.05, that is, a 1 in 20 chance that we conclude there is an association with an exposure and a disease when there is none. The power of a study is the probability of correctly rejecting the null hypothesis. It is related to beta, which is the probability of a type II error, that is, failing to reject the null hypothesis when the null hypothesis is false (power = 1 − beta).

Sample size calculation for case control studies. The number of cases and controls required to investigate the study hypotheses must be calculated before any detailed planning of the study is undertaken. First, it is necessary to decide on the effect size (i.e. odds ratio) that is being investigated. The presumed odds ratio may be based on previous or pilot studies, or a judgement about the size of effect that the investigators consider is of public health or clinical importance to detect. In addition to the odds ratio, other information is required for sample size calculations: the expected prevalence of the exposure in the control population, the number of controls to each case, the alpha level (usually 0.05), and the power of the study (usually 0.8 or above). Information on the expected prevalence of exposure may be available from previous studies or surveys. In this situation where no prior information is available, it will be necessary to carry out a pilot study to obtain this information.

Study power can also be increased by increasing the number of controls per case. This can be considered in situations when it is difficult or expensive to recruit cases. In general, there is little gain in power for increasing the number of controls per case beyond three. The main advantage of doing the sample size calculations as the first step in planning the study is that the information aids the investigator in key design considerations, such as whether to recruit cases from many centres, the time necessary for recruitment of cases and controls, and the decision concerning the number of controls per case (1).

Sample size calculation for randomized controlled trials. For clinical trials designed to detect differences between treatment groups, the number of patients needed for analysis depends on four key quantities:

1. The minimum size of the difference on the primary outcome measure believed to be clinically meaningful.
2. The standard deviation of the primary outcome measure in the patient population to be studied.
3. The type I error level to be used for statistical testing in the final analysis.
4. The desired statistical power to detect the designated difference.

Clinicians and statisticians need to work together because making realistic choices for these quantities often requires judgement and, sometimes, educated guesses.

$$N = \frac{2\left[\left(\frac{Z\alpha}{2} + Z\beta\right)*(SD)\right]^2}{(Difference)^2}$$

4.5 SAMPLING TECHNIQUES

There are two types of sampling in epidemiology:

- Probability sampling
  - Simple random sampling (SRS)
  - Systematic random sampling
  - Cluster sampling (CLS)
  - Multi-phasic sampling

- Non-probability sampling
  - Convenience sampling
  - Purposive sampling
  - Quota sampling
  - Snowball sampling

Although there are numerous techniques of random sampling, the most commonly used in ophthalmic epidemiology is cluster sampling (CLS). In CLS, the population members are divided into non-overlapping groups ("clusters") of individuals, and a sample of the clusters is chosen to yield a sample of the population members. Three main varieties of CLS may be defined, as follows.

One-stage cluster sampling. The population is divided into a number of primary clusters (usually 30 or more), either by census, enumeration areas, neighbourhoods, or villages. Having randomly selected a number of clusters, no further sampling is carried out, and all population members (individuals) within the selected clusters are included in the final sample of individuals. When the clusters have approximately the same number of individuals, SRS is used to draw the sample of clusters, in which case the procedure approximates an equal probability of selection method. When the cluster sizes differ appreciably, the preceding procedure for selecting a sample of clusters is modified to "ensure" equal probability of selection. This involves allocating a proportionally higher probability of selection to clusters that are larger, an important principle known as probability proportional to size (PPS). This is done because most populations are made up of a few large clusters (e.g. towns) and many small clusters (e.g. villages), and if SRS were applied, then all clusters would have an equal chance of being selected, and the selected sample would over-represent people from small clusters and under-represent people from large clusters, compared with the actual population. As the prevalence of a disease may vary between the small and large clusters (e.g. due to access to treatment), this could bias the prevalence estimate. However, statistical methods are available for obtaining unbiased estimates in such situations. Most eye surveys using cluster sampling employ PPS, because in most populations, it is very difficult to define or identify convenient boundaries that delineate groups of equal size.

Two-stage cluster sampling. In this procedure, a number of clusters are selected randomly from the primary clusters (as previously), but within each chosen cluster, only a sample of the individuals is included. As in one-stage CLS, PPS is usually employed to select the clusters, but a fixed (predefined) number of individuals is drawn from every chosen cluster. Selection of individuals within the clusters can be through SRS of all the eligible participants. In this case, the individuals within each chosen cluster are listed in a sampling frame, and a random sample (usually SRS) is drawn from the frame. All the individuals thus selected are included in the final sample. Another frequently used method is the random walk method, where a starting point is defined in the cluster and a bottle is spun to select an arbitrary starting direction. A house in the line of the bottle is chosen, and the enumerators include individuals door to door until the desired cluster size is achieved. There are also variations of the basic random walk method (e.g. choosing consecutive houses at a set interval). There are a number of limitations to the random walk method. This method does not select households from a sampling frame, and so the sample is not selected with a known probability. Furthermore, this method of selection may be open to conscious or unconscious bias of the enumerator in selecting households.

Another method for selecting individuals within clusters is through the compact segment method. In this method, the cluster is divided into areas so that each area includes approximately the same number of people. One of the areas is chosen at random, and either all the participants in that area are included or else a specified number is included (in which case the method would be more like three-stage cluster sampling), and sampling ceases when the required sample size is obtained.

Multi-stage cluster sampling. When the defined population to be sampled is that of a large region or country, it may be more convenient (logistically and for economy) to group the population members first in large clusters (called primary sampling units, or PSU) that may correspond to, for example, districts or states. Within each PSU, the individuals are grouped into a number of smaller convenient clusters (second-stage units). These subunits may be administrative divisions within the PSU (e.g. blocks). Yet smaller subgroups of individuals may be defined within each second-stage unit (e.g. enumeration units in trachoma surveys), and so on. Selecting first from among PSUs, then from secondary units within selected PSUs, and then within the secondary units, and so on generates the sample. This method of sampling enables a representative sample to be obtained across provinces so that the sample may be more generalizable.

4.6 RAPID ASSESSMENT METHODS IN COMMUNITY OPHTHALMOLOGY

The Rapid Assessment of Avoidable Blindness (RAAB) is a survey design using CLS sampling to achieve the desired sample size. It was developed by Hans Limburg as a simple and rapid survey methodology to provide data on the prevalence and causes of blindness and is a modified version of the RACSS (2). A RAAB is ideally carried out at the level of a district or province that has a population size of 0.5 to 5 million people. The sample size required for a RAAB is usually between 2,000 and 5,000 people but depends on the expected prevalence of blindness and the desired precision of the estimate. Clusters of people to include in the survey are randomly selected from across the survey area through PPS. Each day, a team visits one population unit (preferably an enumeration area used by the census office, which a is small, clearly demarcated area with a known population often corresponding to a village or suburb of a town). Individuals within the cluster are selected through a modification of compact segment sampling. The cluster is divided into geographical units each including approximately 50 people aged 50+, and one segment is randomly selected. The team then goes to the selected area and visits the households door to door until they have enumerated 50 people aged over 50 years (the cluster). All selected people undergo visual acuity screening with a tumbling E chart and have their lenses examined. The main cause of VA < 6/18 is determined by an ophthalmologist or ophthalmic clinical officer. The information collected in the RAAB is used to estimate the prevalence of blindness in the survey area, taking into account the design effect, and causes of blindness are also estimated. Data from RAAB can also be used to assess outcomes after cataract surgery, barriers to cataract surgery, and cataract surgical coverage.

4.7 DEVELOPING ONLINE DATA COLLECTION TOOLS

These days, several options are available for electronic data collection (EDC) in research projects. EDC can be done using laptops or, more commonly, using smartphones. There are some well-known software, such as Google Forms, SurveyMonkey, etc., which enable the creation of online forms using drag-and-drop interfaces. These are well suited for online surveys and in situations where the data collection form is simple. Software that has been developed specifically for research use include OpenDatKit (ODK), RedCap, EpiCollect, KoboCollect, etc. Standardized surveys, such as RAAB and the Global Trachoma Mapping Project (GTMP), offer custom-built EDC software (mRAAB) that can be licensed for use in eye health surveys.

The most important advantage of using EDC is minimization of data entry or transcription errors when doing data entry after paper-based data collection. Data quality can be ensured at source (during interview or examination) by using rules of allowed values, minimum-maximum, decimals, etc.

Since data entry after paper-based data collection is not needed, time gets saved. By using speech-to-text features available in Android and iOS phone keyboards, the need for typing in responses for qualitative questions can also be reduced. These contribute to improved efficiency and may reduce costs in the conduct of research work.

EDC software include features such as conditional showing or hiding of questions, branching logic, repeatable sections within a form, relational forms, reading barcodes, capturing signatures, GPS coordinates, images, videos, automatic time-stamping, etc. Thus, richer information can be collected.

An important consideration when using electronic data collection is ensuring data security, confidentiality, and backups. Monitoring also becomes trickier as the supervising teams which normally could just pick up completed paper forms for re-verification now need to be given access to completed electronic records, which may not be easy in many EDC systems.

Many of these tools (ODK, RedCap) can be set up for free on a server within the research team, provided the necessary hardware (server, network, etc.) and expertise are available. Another option is to use cloud-based tools, where payments may be required for licensing, but upfront infrastructure costs can be saved. EDC does require initial familiarity with the systems and may involve additional training of research teams, and the team may need to include computer professionals, procurement of computers, software licensing costs, smartphones, etc., leading to increased costs. However, in most instances, these can be offset through time saved with increased efficiency. Overall, EDCs are being increasingly utilized in large-scale as well as small-scale surveys and must be considered seriously for research data collection, due to the numerous advantages they offer.

4.8 CONCLUSION

In this chapter, we have learned about the basic steps in conducting epidemiological research study, sample size calculations, and electronic data collection methods. The underlying philosophy is that if sound, high-quality research methodology is adopted, it is likely to yield results that are reliable and robust.

REFERENCES

1. World Health Organization. Regional Office for the Western Pacific. Health Research Methodology: A Guide for Training in Research Methods Second Edition [Internet]. WHO Regional Office for the Western Pacific; 2001 [cited 2023 Mar 3]. ix, 237 p. Available from: https://apps.who.int/iris/handle/10665/206929
2. Mactaggart, I., Limburg, H., Bastawrous, A., Burton, M. J. & Kuper, H. Rapid Assessment of Avoidable Blindness: Looking Back, Looking Forward. Br. J. Ophthalmol. 103, 1549–1552 (2019).

5

National Programme for Control of Blindness and Visual Impairment

SOUVIK MANNA, PRAVEEN VASHIST, NOOPUR GUPTA

5.1 INTRODUCTION

India was one of the first countries to have a national programme for the control of blindness (now NPCB&VI) in 1976. In 1971–1974, the Indian Council of Medical Research (ICMR) conducted a nationwide survey, and prevalence of blindness was 1.38% (presenting visual acuity < 6/60 in the better eye). The goal of the programme was to reduce the prevalence of blindness to 0.3% initially by the year 2020 and later extended to 2020 (1). The programme superseded the National Trachoma Control Program that was operational since 1963. The programme has been renamed in the year 2017 as the National Programme for Control of Blindness and Visual Impairment (NPCB&VI) (2). The Rapid Survey on Avoidable Blindness conducted under NPCB during 2006–2007 showed reduction in the prevalence of blindness from 1.1% (2001–2002) to 1% (2006–2007) (3). The current prevalence of blindness is 0.36% as per RAAB survey 2015–2019, resulting in 47.1% relative reduction in blindness and 51.9% reduction in VI in 2019 compared to 2010 (4).

Main Objectives of the Programme

- To reduce the backlog of avoidable blindness through identification and treatment of curable blindness at primary, secondary, and tertiary levels, based on assessment of the burden of visual impairment in the country.
- To develop and strengthen the strategy of NPCB&VI for "Eye Health for All" and to prevent visual impairment through the provision of comprehensive universal eye care services and quality service delivery.

- To strengthen and upgrade Regional Institutes of Ophthalmology (RIOs) to become centres of excellence (COE) in various sub-specialties of ophthalmology, and also other partners, like government medical colleges, district hospitals, sub-district hospitals, and vision centres.
- To strengthen the existing infrastructure facilities and develop additional human resources for providing high-quality comprehensive eye care in all districts of the country.
- To enhance community awareness on eye care and lay stress on preventive measures.
- To increase and expand research for prevention of blindness and visual impairment.
- To secure participation of voluntary organizations/non-governmental organizations/private practitioners in delivering eye care services.

Programme Objectives Are to be Achieved by Adopting the Following Strategy

- Decentralized implementation of the scheme through district health societies of blindness.
- Reduction in the backlog of blind persons by active screening of population above 50 years, organizing screening eye camps, and transporting operable cases to fixed eye care facilities.
- Involvement of voluntary organizations in various eye care activities.
- Ensuring participation of community and Panchayati Raj institutions (PRI) in organizing services in rural areas.
- Development of eye care services and improvement in quality of eye care by training of personnel, supply of high-tech ophthalmic equipment, strengthening follow-up services, and regular monitoring of services.
- Screening of school children (primary and secondary) for identification and treatment of refractive errors, with special attention in underserved areas.
- Public awareness about prevention and timely treatment of common eye ailments.
- Special focus on illiterate women in rural areas. For this purpose, there should be convergence with various ongoing schemes for development.
- Treatment of cataract and other eye diseases, like diabetic retinopathy, glaucoma management, corneal transplantation, vitreoretinal surgery, treatment of childhood blindness, etc.
- Construction of dedicated eye wards and eye OTs in district hospitals in NE states and few other states as per need.
- Development of mobile ophthalmic units in NE states and other hilly states linked with teleophthalmic network and few fixed models.
- Involvement of private practitioners in the sub-district, blocks, and village levels.

The programme extends assistance to non-government organizations (NGO) for providing eye care services, including cataract operations and eye banking.

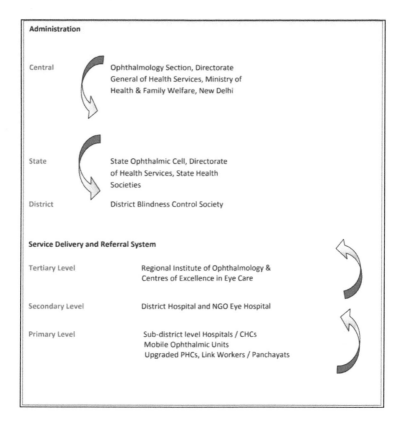

Figure 5.1 Organogram of NPCB&VI

NGOs play an important role in this programme. District Blindness Control Societies (DBCS), as part of district health societies for decentralized programme management, have been established throughout the country under the chairmanship of the district collector/deputy commissioner (5). Apart from cataract surgeries, now the focus of the programme is on treatment and management of other eye diseases, like glaucoma, diabetic retinopathy, vitreoretinal diseases, corneal blindness, low vision, and childhood blindness. The programme is now geared to take care of all categories of visual impairment. Under the national programme, some of the tertiary care centres were upgraded to centres of excellence (Regional Institutes of Ophthalmology [RIO]), focusing on the development of manpower and infrastructure. In order to facilitate the outreach activities, more than 3,000 vision centres were started in providing primary eye care services. These peripheral vision centres, staffed with a trained ophthalmic assistant, can carry out comprehensive eye examination and management of simple eye diseases. Currently, the plan is to establish vision centres at the level of community health centres (secondary-level health centres), later scaling up to the primary health centre level.

India has implemented a series of measures in its ongoing National Programme for Control of Blindness and Visual Impairment (NPCB&VI) to combat blindness and visual impairment in the country. About 65% of surgical performance in the country is performed in the private and voluntary sector, and only 35% is within the government sector. About 21,000 ophthalmologists exist in India.

5.2 A PATTERN OF ASSISTANCE

The pattern of assistance during the three-year period (2017–2020) is given here:

- NPCB&VI would be part of the NCD Flexible Pool under the overarching umbrella of the National Health Mission (NHM). Funds for implementation of the programme would be released by NHM through the respective state health societies in the form of grant-in-aid into the NPCB&VI account.
- Assistance for performing free cataract surgeries with intraocular lens (IOL) implantation by NGOs and private practitioners.
- Assistance to government hospitals for performing cataract surgeries, etc., towards drugs and surgical consumables, like visco-elastics, blades, fluids, etc.
- In addition to cataract, assistance for other eye diseases, like diabetic retinopathy, glaucoma management, treatment of childhood blindness, corneal transplantation, and vitreoretinal surgery to, NGOs and private practitioners.
- Assistance to eye banks and eye donation centres for improvement in cornea collection and eye banking services.
- Assistance for construction of dedicated eye units in district hospitals in NE states and few other states as per need.
- Engagement of manpower, such as ophthalmic surgeons, donation counsellors, and data entry operators at district level on contractual basis to meet the shortage of manpower in states.
- Assistance for maintenance of ophthalmic equipment supplied under the programme.
- Assistance for multipurpose district mobile ophthalmic units (MDMOU) to improve coverage.
- Assistance for setting up of fixed teleophthalmology network units in government set-up with linkage to ophthalmic consultation units through the internet, intensification of IEC activities.
- Strengthening of management information system (MIS) and release of funds to NGOs/private practitioners on the basis of the entries in NPCB-MIS and verification of 5% cases.

NPCB&VI would be part of the NCD Flexible Pool under the overarching umbrella of the National Health Mission (NHM). The following decisions have been taken to streamline the working of state health societies/district health societies (blindness).

All work related to blindness control in state will be routed through the state programme officer/joint director (ophthalmology) in charge of NPCB&VI, while the state programme officer/joint director shall submit it to the director of Health Services for final approval in accordance with the approved pattern of assistance. All the state PIPs for blindness control shall be prepared in accordance with the guidelines issued by the centre and in consultation with the programme division at the centre. The state government/UT administration will not divert/alter any component or part(s) without the approval of the programme division of the MoH&FW. It will be the responsibility of the state government/UT administration to submit the utilization certificate within the prescribed time period to settle the grant released under the programme as per the approved financial norm of GoI.

Attention is also invited towards provision for appointment of contractual manpower in state in the duration of years 2017–2020. State government/UT administrations are requested to take advance action for making provisions for inclusion of necessary ophthalmic manpower in state/UT's budget after completion of the three-year period in March 2020. The central government will not be responsible for the salary, etc., of the contractual manpower in case the scheme is discontinued. This pattern of assistance for the three-year period (2017–2020) will be effective World Economic Forum (WEF) financial year 2018–2019.

5.3 PATTERN OF ASSISTANCE UNDER NPCB&VI

Table 5.1 Pattern of Assistance under NPCB&VI

Component Recurring Grant-in-Aid	Pattern of Assistance during 2017–2020
Grant-in-aid for cataract operations in government sector and NGO/private sector	Reimbursement for cataract operation for NGOs and private practitioners (@ Rs. 2,000/case.
	Assistance for cataract operations for government sector @ Rs. 1,000/case.
	In cases where NGOs/private practitioners are using government OT: a. Normal area: **@ Rs. 1,200/**case. b. Difficult areas, such as tribal, desert, hilly, and north-eastern districts: **@ Rs. 2,000/**case.
	For identifying blind persons (blind registry), organizing and motivating identified persons, and transporting them to government/VC fixed facilities for cataract surgeries, panchayats, ICDS functionaries. ASHA workers, and other voluntary groups like mahila mandals would be identified and involved by the district health societies. They would be eligible for support not exceeding Rs. 350/operated case (if the patient is transported to the NGO facility for surgery, Rs 350 shall be paid by the NGO out of Rs. 2,000 which it received as reimbursement for any free cataract surgery performed).

Continued

Table 5.1 Continued

Grant-in-aid for treatment/ management of other eye diseases to NGOs and private practitioners	Diabetic retinopathy @ **Rs. 2,000**; childhood blindness @ **Rs. 2,000**; glaucoma @ **pRs. 2,000**; keratoplasty @ **SPRs. 7,500**; vitreoretinal surgery @ Rs. 10,000.
Grant-in-aid for distribution of free spectacles to schoolchildren to district health societies	Screening and free spectacles to schoolchildren @ **Rs. 350/spectacles.**
Grant-in-aid for distribution of free spectacles to elderly population to district health societies	Screening and free spectacles for near work to old persons @ **Rs. 350/spectacles.**
Grant-in-aid to eye banks in government/ voluntary sector	Recurring GIA to eye bank @ **Rs. 2,000/pair** of eyes (eye bank will reimburse to eye donation centre attached with it for eye collected by them @ **Rs. 1,000/pair of** eyes) to meet the cost of consumables, including preservation material and media, transportation/POL, and contingencies.
Grant-in-aid for training of PMOAs and other paramedics	The trainings PMOAs and other paramedics will be conducted at state/district level as per the NHM norms.
Grant-in-aid for Information, education, and communication (IEC) in state/district	**State-level IEC @ Rs. 10 lakh** for minor states and **Rs. 20 lakh** for major states. State-**level activities:** for development of IEC strategy in various regions of the state, replication of effective prototype, monitoring of district-level IEC activities. **District-level activities:** local IEC suitable to target population, use of folk methods, and other indigenous means of communication, orientation of local leaders, etc.
Grant-in-aid for maintenance of ophthalmic equipment	Maintenance of ophthalmic equipment @ **pRs. 5 lakh/ district** to ensure longevity of costly ophthalmic equipment supplied under the programme. (States shall include this activity in biomedical equipment maintenance programme (BEMP. However, the state may continue the existing procedure till the activity is awarded under BEMP.)

Table 5.1 Continued

Management of state health society	Up to **Rs. 20 lakh** to meet expenditure on the following activities:
	1. Staff
	  a. Budget finance officer—as proposed by state
	  b. Administrative assistant—preferably through outsourced mode
	  c. MTS—preferably through outsourced mode
	  d. Data entry operations—to be decided on the programme workload
	2. Other expenses
	  a. Mobility support, review meetings, etc.

Grant-in-aid for district hospitals/sub-district hospitals/vision centres	Strengthening of district hospitals/sub-district hospitals/PHCs (vision centres) in government sector (as per IPHS norms based on the state proposals). (The list of ophthalmic equipment for district hospitals/sub-district hospitals/ vision centres will be provided with detailed guidelines.)
Grant-in-aid for eye banks	Eye banks in public sector up to **Rs. 40 lakh per unit** for equipment and furnishing towards strengthening/ developing eye banks. (The list of equipment, instruments, etc. for eye banks will be provided with detailed guidelines.)
Grant-in-aid for eye donation centres	Eye donation centre in public sector up to Rs. 1 lakh/ unit for strengthening/developing eye donation centre.
Grant-in-aid for construction of dedicated eye units	Construction of dedicated eye unit (eye ward and eye OT) in public sector @ **Rs. 100 lakh**/unit.
Grant-in-aid for procurement of multipurpose district mobile ophthalmic unit with equipment	Procurement of Multipurpose Distt. Mobile ophthalmic Unit with equipments. Operating cost, including salary, maintenance, and POL, etc., @ Rs. 30 lakh/unit.
Grant-in-aid for tele-network	Approximate cost of a tele-network unit @ **Rs. 25** lakh/unit (4–5 vision centres to be linked to district hospital/medical college/tertiary care centre, whichever is nearer).
Component: Contractual Manpower	**Pattern of Assistance during 2017–2020**

Continued

Table 5.1 Continued

Grant-in-aid for contractual manpower	1. Ophthalmic surgeon in district hospitals.* 2. Ophthalmic assistant in PHC/vision centres, district hospitals, and sub-district hospitals.* 3. Eye donation counsellors in eye banks.* 4. Data entry operator at district level (to be decided on the basis of programme workload).

*As per IPHS norms based on the state proposals.

REFERENCES

1. Directorate General of Health Services [Internet]. [cited 2020 May 27]. Available from: https://dghs.gov.in/content/1354_3_NationalProgrammeforControlofBlindnessVisual.aspx
2. Ministry of Health and Family Welfare. Operational Guidelines Eye Care at Health and Wellness Centres (Part of Comprehensive Primary Health Care). 2019. Pp. 1–20. Available from: https://ab-hwc.nhp.gov.in/
3. National Program for Control of Blindness & Visual Impairment [Internet]. [cited 2020 Jan 16]. Available from: https://npcbvi.gov.in/Home
4. Vashist P, Senjam SS, Gupta V, Gupta N, Shamanna BR, Wadhwani M, Shukla P, Manna S, Yadav S, Bharadwaj A. Blindness and visual impairment and their causes in India: Results of a nationally representative survey. PLoS One. 2022 Jul;17(7):e0271736.
5. Jose R, Bachani D. World bank-assisted cataract blindness control project. Indian J Ophthalmol. 1995 Jan 1;43(1):35–43.

6

Vision 2020: The Right to Sight

A Global Initiative to Effectively Address Blindness and Visual Impairment

PHANINDRA BABU NUKELLA, PRAVEEN VASHIST

6.1 CONTEXT

The World Health Assembly, in 1975, adopted a resolution requesting the director-general to act against the problem of blindness and to establish initiatives against trachoma, xerophthalmia, cataract, onchocerciasis, ocular trauma, and glaucoma. Following this resolution, the World Health Organization (WHO) Programme for the Prevention of Blindness was officially established in Geneva in 1978.

In line with this commitment, the International Agency for the Prevention of Blindness (IAPB) was established in 1975 by the International Council of Ophthalmology and the World Blind Union. IAPB was established as a coordinating umbrella organization to lead an international effort in mobilizing resources for blindness prevention activities. IAPB links national programs for the prevention of blindness, non-governmental organizations (NGOs), educational institutions, individuals, and the founding organizations. In addition, IAPB has an official relationship with the WHO Programme on Prevention of Blindness and Deafness based in Geneva, Switzerland, and with the blindness prevention coordinator assigned to some WHO regional offices.

6.2 VISION 2020 GLOBAL

Vision 2020: The Right to Sight, the global initiative for the elimination of avoidable blindness by the year 2020, was formally launched on 18 February 1999 by the World Health Organization and the International Agency for the Prevention of Blindness.

DOI: 10.1201/9781003291626-6

> **It sought to promote:**
> "A world in which nobody is needlessly visually impaired, where those with unavoidable vision loss can achieve their full potential."
>
> **The Global Initiative was set up to:**
> "Intensify and accelerate prevention of blindness activities so as to achieve the goal of eliminating avoidable blindness by 2020."
>
> **It sought to do this by:**
> "Focusing initially on certain diseases which are the main causes of blindness and for which proven cost effective interventions are available."

In May 2003, the WHO Resolution on Elimination of Avoidable Blindness was adopted by the 56th World Health Assembly, which calls on all member states to commit themselves to Vision 2020 plans by 2005. Considering various studies and publications, the IAPB 2010 report was launched to mark the halfway point of the goals of Vision 2020.

6.3 RECENT DEVELOPMENTS: WORLD HEALTH ASSEMBLY RESOLUTIONS

Four World Health Assembly resolutions (2003, 2006, 2009, and 2013) reinforced the aim and objectives of Vision 2020. The last two resolutions were accompanied by WHO action plans which provided more detail on how the objectives were to be achieved. They also helped refine some of the implementation approaches.

The "Universal Eye Health: A Global Action Plan 2014–2019" (GAP) was unanimously adopted by member states at the World Health Assembly in 2013 as part of WHA Resolution 66.4. The plan, building upon and replacing previous Vision 2020 and 2009–2013 action plans, committed governments to a 25% reduction in the prevalence of avoidable visual impairment by the year 2019 from the baseline of 2010.

A 2020 World Health Assembly resolution urges **integrated people-centred eye care** to be embedded, within the principal health agenda of universal health coverage and to expand the scope of eye care into the mainstream as an integral issue for sustainable development.

6.4 GLOBAL COMMITMENTS TO EYE HEALTH AND UNIVERSAL HEALTH COVERAGE

1. **United Nations Political Declaration**
   The IAPB, together with the United Nations Friends of Vision, successfully advocated for the inclusion of eye health in the first political declaration of the high-level meeting on universal health coverage. Heads of states committed to strengthen efforts to address eye health conditions as part of UHC. This is an important milestone for the global eye health community, as it recognizes that UHC cannot be achieved without eye health.

2. **World Health Assembly Resolution on Integrated People-Centred Eye Care**
   The commitment was further strengthened by a World Health Assembly resolution on integrated people-centred eye care. The resolution requires all countries to make eye care an integral part of universal health coverage and to implement the recommendations of the World Report on Vision, specifically to integrate people-centred eye care into their national health systems.

3. **World Health Assembly Global Targets on Eye Health**
   Two new ambitious eye health targets for 2030 were adopted at the 74th World Health Assembly. The targets address the two leading causes of blindness and vision impairment, cataract and refractive error, and are a vital mechanism to monitor global progress on eye health and to hold governments accountable.
   To address the huge unmet need in eye care, all countries have committed to:
   - 40% increase in effective coverage of refractive error (eREC) by 2030
   - 30% increase in effective coverage of cataract surgery (eCSC) by 2030

eCSC is defined as the proportion of people who have received cataract surgery and have a resultant good quality outcome (6/12 or better) relative to the number of people in need of cataract surgery.

eREC is defined as the proportion of people who have received refractive error services (that is, spectacles, contact lenses, or refractive surgery) and have a resultant good quality outcome relative to the number of people in need of refractive error services.

The latest tools developed by the WHO to support universal eye health include:

1. *Package of eye care interventions (PECI).* Includes evidence-based and cost-effective eye care interventions and approaches to facilitate the integration of eye care into universal health coverage across the continuum of (a) health promotion and prevention, (b) screening, (c) diagnosis and monitoring, (d) treatment, and (e) rehabilitation. The interventions are also presented across the life course, that is, which intervention should be done in children, adolescents, adults, or all age groups and how they link out to other health programs, such as maternal and newborn health, school health, non-communicable disease control, etc. (1).

2. *Eye care competency framework (ECCF).* Competencies are the ability of individuals to carry out activities and express behaviours, using their knowledge and skills. The ECCF includes the knowledge and skills that eye care workers should have to effectively deliver quality and integrated eye care services across primary to tertiary levels of healthcare (2).

3. *Eye care indicator menu (ECIM).* Provides a list of input, output, outcome, and impact indicators from which countries can select to facilitate the monitoring of strategies and actions for eye care at national and subnational level (3).

4. *Eye care in health systems.* A guide to help countries analyze, plan, implement, and review integrated people-centred eye care (IPEC) in their own
healthcare systems. It lists the steps and activities required for situation
analysis, development of eye care strategic plans, monitoring framework, and
operational plans for implementation of the strategic plan (4).

6.5 VISION 2020: THE RIGHT TO SIGHT, INDIA

Respecting the sanctity and commitment of the WHO resolution of May 2003,
and following the earlier discussions, **Vision 2020: The Right to Sight, India**
(Vision 2020 India), was set up by nine founding members (non-governmental organizations engaged in eye care) in the year 2004. The forum is a collaborative effort of international NGOs, NGO eye care organizations, and
Dr RP Centre of Ophthalmic Sciences, AIIMS, and eye care industry in India
to coordinate and support for improved eye care programmes, gaining and
sharing knowledge and thinking solutions together to achieve quality, comprehensive, and equitable eye care. The primary objective of Vision 2020
India is to "intensify and accelerate prevention of blindness activities so as
to achieve the goal of eliminating avoidable blindness through policy environment and strengthening the capacity of eye care institutions." It is a key
driver of the joint global initiative of the World Health Organization (WHO)
and International Agency for the Prevention of Blindness (IAPB) for reducing
avoidable visual impairment.

Under the global initiative, in 2012, the 9th General Assembly in Hyderabad
attracted 1,600 delegates from 86 countries, doubling the numbers of previous
assemblies. The assembly culminated with the endorsement by acclamation of the
Hyderabad Declaration, calling on international organizations, regional entities,
governments, civil society, and the private sector to work together to ensure that
blindness and visual impairment are adequately and comprehensively addressed
within an inclusive international development framework and as part of primary
healthcare and health systems. This further reinforced the aims and mission of
Vision 2020 India and led to developing its own five-year strategic plans guiding
its roadmap in country context.

Vision of Vision 2020 India

- India free of avoidable blindness, where every citizen enjoys the gift of sight
and the visually challenged have enhanced quality of life as a right.

Mission of Vision 2020 India

- Work with eye care organizations in India for the elimination of avoidable
blindness by provision of equitable and affordable services as well as rehabilitation of visually challenged persons.

Policy advocacy, strengthening eye care, and organizational development of its own and of its members have remained as the three core focus areas for Vision 2020 India.

6.6 KEY CONTRIBUTIONS TO SUPPORT AND COMPLEMENT THE NATIONAL PROGRAMME

- *Guidelines for the management of Cataract in India*, published in the year 2020, incorporating Covid context. Reviewed by DDG (O), NPCB&VI, and developed by a technical committee including Dr RP Centre, AIIMS. This document would be very useful at the time when the government launched cataract blindness backlog–free initiative across the country. This document sets systems, protocols, and good practices for an effective cataract surgery. The previous version of this document was referred by the state governments of Punjab, Chandigarh, and West Bengal on certain occasions.
- *Developed Arunachal Pradesh State eye health action plan.* Vision 2020 India developed eye health action plan for Arunachal Pradesh in the year 2016. This led to public–private partnerships (PPP) in Arunachal, and such partnerships helped the state declare few villages cataract blindness backlog–free, and the capacity of local healthcare workers (ASHAs) improved, coupled with renovated OT in a CHC. The whole eye care service delivery and training gained momentum in the state.
- *Cataract backlog–free district.* Partners of Vision 2020 India (like Sadguru Netra Chikitsalaya, Chitrakoot) demonstrated that a cataract blindness backlog–free district can be achieved and created its own model. It further encouraged other stakeholders in the country to move forward with that spirit and make more districts cataract blindness backlog–free. Moving ahead, the NPCB&VI also launched a scheme of cataract blindness backlog–free districts/states with a financial incentive in year 2020.
- *Increase in grant-in-aid (GiA) for NGOs.* In 2017, Vision 2020 India discussed with the then joint secretary of NPCB&VI to consider increasing grant-in-aid for NGOs, providing the rationale of increased unit costs incurred by NPCB&VI partner hospitals. The increase took place; for example, cataract GiA was increased from Rs. 1,000 to Rs. 2,000/case, and so on for other eye conditions. NPCB&VI partner hospitals were happy and complementing the national programme.

6.7 STRATEGIC PLAN, MEMBERSHIP, AND GOVERNANCE

Vision 2020 India's strategic plan for 2016–2021 has been developed to achieve the mission and vision of the organization. It involves a considerable volume of work of analyzing the success of the previous one and then building upon that. It was made possible due to the valuable time and feedback and suggestions given by various stakeholders. It includes five objectives:

1. **Universalize.** Demonstrate universal eye health coverage with integrated people-centred eye care, with a focus on primary eye care, including specific target populations, and with the specific intention of ensuring equity.
2. **Consolidate.** Demonstrate consolidation of resources for effective policy implementation of eye care through government community health centres, primary health centres, health and wellness centres, and ASHAs.
3. **Systematize.** Design and develop a comprehensive, community-based health management information system (HMIS) which facilitates early detection of eye health needs, planning at all levels, implementation, and monitoring of integrated population-based eye health services in a defined population. To generate demand for eye care service and modify service utilization behaviours and strengthen primary care services through telecommunication and technology.
4. **Coordinate.** Bring together the diverse members of the Vision 2020 India network into a harmonious and efficient relationship with each other and with officials of the central and state governments and industry in order to achieve synchronous and synergistic outcomes.
5. **Advocate.** Undertake policy advocacy at the level of both central and state governments, enable the advancement of innovations being undertaken in the non-government sector's influence shifts in policy formulation and its implementation, and provide evidence through evaluations and multi-centric research to support the policy addressal of eye care needs and replication of best practices.

6.8 GOVERNANCE

The board of management provides oversight and meets each quarter to review the performance. The organization follows standard systems and protocols for financial management and programme management. Also, each year, the general body meets, reviews programme plans and achievements, and ratifies decisions. The executive committee meets each month and reviews performance and takes certain decisions. Six zones represent the country operations, and each zone has one zonal representative on the board, in addition to a national coordinator.

REFERENCES

1. World Health Organization. Package of eye care interventions [Internet]. World Health Organization; 2022 [cited 2023 Mar 3]. x, 99 p. Available from: https://apps.who.int/iris/handle/10665/354256
2. World Health Organization. Eye care competency framework [Internet]. World Health Organization; 2022 [cited 2023 Mar 3]. viii, 68 p. Available from: https://apps.who.int/iris/handle/10665/354241

3. World Health Organization. Eye care indicator menu (ECIM): a tool for monitoring strategies and actions for eye care provision [Internet]. World Health Organization; 2022 [cited 2023 Mar 3]. vi, 46 p. Available from: https://apps.who.int/iris/handle/10665/354257

4. World Health Organization. Eye care in health systems: guide for action [Internet]. World Health Organization; 2022 [cited 2023 Mar 3]. vi, 62 p. Available from: https://apps.who.int/iris/handle/10665/354382

7

Primary Eye Care and Practices

PALLAVI SHUKLA, MEERA SHARMA, PRAVEEN VASHIST

7.1 DEFINING PRIMARY EYE CARE

Primary eye care is a frontline activity providing eye care and disease identification before it becomes serious (1). The purpose is to make eye care services available, accessible, acceptable, and affordable to the masses. It is an integral part of comprehensive eye care capturing the entire spectrum of prevention right from primary, secondary, to rehabilitative care. It provides a person not only with the first point of contact for eye care but also with a continuum of care across life course. It is thus imperative to maintain the quality and sustainability of these services.

7.2 NEED FOR PRIMARY EYE CARE

As is depicted in the World Report on Vision, "everyone will experience at least one eye condition in their lifetime provided they live for so long" (2). If people visit tertiary hospitals for minor ocular ailments, the hospitals shall be overburdened and those in need for specialist treatment shall have to wait in endless queues.

There are around 2.2 billion people who are living with vision impairment. Among these cases, around 1 billion vision impairment could have been prevented (2). These preventable conditions could have easily been managed with appropriate primary care and timely referral.

Age, gender, geographic locations, rural–urban divide are few variables which impact the accessibility of health services. Primary eye care is also needed to mitigate the inequities in accessing eye care services.

7.3 ESSENTIALS OF PRIMARY EYE CARE (3)

The basic primary eye care package comprises of:

Awareness generation. Generating awareness in community about eye conditions leading to visual impairment and those eye conditions which cause

 DOI: 10.1201/9781003291626-7

discomfort to the patient. This would lead to increase in demand generation for eye care services. By educating people about the myths and barriers
associated with several eye diseases, the apprehension associated with it can
be mitigated and accessibility enhanced.

Basic ophthalmic examination. Provision for a basic ophthalmic examination
needed to make certain definitive diagnoses, like conjunctivitis, cataract,
refractive error, and certain probable diagnoses, like diabetic retinopathy,
trachoma, glaucoma, globe abnormalities, etc.

Screening for asymptomatic eye diseases and conditions affecting vision.
Provision for opportunistic eye examination to one and all visiting the health
facility for any other non-ophthalmic illness. Sometimes, even in the absence
of symptoms, person may be harbouring an eye condition which could cause
gradual diminution of vision, like cataract, open-angle glaucoma, etc.

Performing refractions. This is the key ingredient of primary eye care recipe.
Refractive error is the most common visual concern of the people and also an
important cause of visual impairment. This is one component which can correct
the condition completely at the primary level. It has to be linked with the availability of good-quality, low-cost optical aids, like glasses and contact lenses.

Referral linkages. Appropriate referral mechanism needs to be in place. Timely
referral is crucial for saving as well as restoring eyesight. Referral also
includes back referrals. Those are patients referred to higher centres who
need to be tracked back to primary level to ensure their follow-up and compliance to treatment, especially in chronic eye conditions and post-operative
cases. Referral management also includes referral from community by community volunteers.

Patient education and counselling. A primary physician/primary health
worker's job does not end at examination and prescription. They need to
invest quality time in educating patient about his/her eye condition and
how it shall be managed at all levels. Proper counselling by these primary
workers goes a long way in ensuring proper follow-up and compliance to
treatment.

***Coordinating care with other physicians involved in the patient's overall medical
management.*** There are certain systemic diseases which have ocular manifes-
tation. Likewise, certain ocular medications lead to systemic manifestations.
Primary eye care workers should be working in close contact with primary
physicians. Therefore, eye care services integrated with primary healthcare
facility could be helpful in overall patient management.

7.4 LEVELS OF EYE CARE DELIVERY IN INDIA

Before delving into levels of eye care, it's important to know the public health infrastructure of India. The healthcare facilities are categorized as:

1. *Sub-centre (SC).* Peripheral outpost of a primary health centre (PHC), catering to a population of 3,000 to 5,000. It is staffed with one auxiliary nurse
midwife (ANM) and one health worker (male). Services provided at SC are

mostly promotive and preventive, with some curative component. These sub-centres are linked with the community through ground-level volunteers, like accredited social health activists (ASHA).

2. *Primary health centre (PHC).* Catering to a population of 20,000 to 30,000. This centre is staffed with a medical officer, auxiliary nurse midwife, lab technician, pharmacist, and lady health visitor. It provides for outpatient services, 24-hour emergency services, and limited inpatient care pertaining to maternal and child health, including deliveries.

3. *Community health centre (CHC).* Facility catering to a population of 80,000 to 1.20 lakh with 30 beds and availability of specialists in various fields, like gynaecology, paediatrics, medicine, and surgery, and provision for X-ray and laboratory services. It provides for the entire package of reproductive, maternal, and child healthcare, including 24-hour delivery services, essential newborn care, and routine and emergency care of sick newborn. Staff at CHC include specialist doctors from surgery, medicine, gynaecology, and paediatrics, dental surgeon, ophthalmologist, anaesthetist, public health manager, AYUSH doctors, staff nurses, pharmacists, lab technicians, and other support staff.

4. *Hospitals.* It includes sub-district, district hospitals, and medical colleges. There is a difference between "health centre" and "hospital" wherein the former provides only curative care and the latter provides a spectrum of promotive, preventive, and curative care. Hospital does not have boundaries, whereas centre has defined population and defined area.

This was the basic public health infrastructure in India.

7.5 PYRAMIDAL MODEL OF EYE CARE IN INDIA

The model was first developed by LV Prasad Eye Institute, and the same was adopted by Vision 2020: Right to Sight India (4). It included a four-tiered pyramid of eye care facilities. Recently, a fifth tier has been added. At the apex are the centres of excellence, which are around 20 in number; their main purpose is research, training, and capacity building of all other lower centres. Below them lie the tertiary care centres, serving a population of 5 million. These centres are well equipped for complex, sophisticated, and advance eye care services. Right below them under tertiary centres are the service centres, catering to a population of 5 lakhs. These centres provide comprehensive ophthalmic examination and basic ophthalmic surgeries like for cataract. The fourth tier is the vision centre. It's a fixed-facility primary-level centre for eye care manned by an ophthalmic assistant and well connected to the base hospitals, which are either service centres or tertiary centres. This vision centre serves a population of 50,000. Primary centres are suited to the basic need of the community and should be as close to the people as possible. However, at times, even the availability of these services does not ensure its utilization. In order to improve the accessibility of these centres, it was thought to connect them to the community through grassroots-level volunteers, like vision

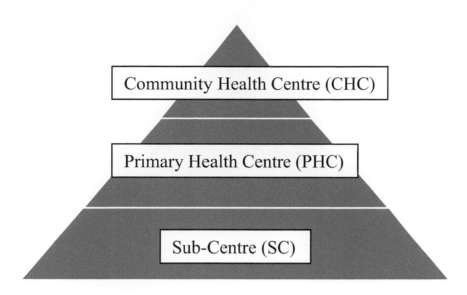

Figure 7.1 Various levels of eye care.

guardians of LVPEI. This accounts for the bottom-most tiers. Each vision guardian looks after a community of 5,000 people.

The model was successfully adopted by LVPEI in a standalone fashion. However, the model needs to be integrated in the public health system for a better penetration across the length and breadth of India.

7.6 INTEGRATED PEOPLE-CENTRED EYE CARE

The World Report on Vision sets out concrete proposals to address challenges in eye care. The key proposal is to make integrated people-centred eye care embedded in health systems. It should be based on the principles of strong primary health-care, the care model of choice, and scale it up widely. Eye care is often considered specialist care and is not available at the community level. Eye conditions are very common, and some of them may even turn to be sight-threatening if not managed in crucial time. Unavailability of basic eye care services near to the people might create a huge gap in optimum service utilization.

The stage is set for integrated eye care. The public health infrastructure of India is in a state of reform with the advent of the Ayushman Bharat scheme and the development of health and wellness centres. The plans have been formulated to strengthen primary eye care (PEC). This PEC shall be provided at these three levels:

1. Vision centres at the level of existing CHCs
2. Health and wellness centres at the level of PHCs
3. Community level through grassroots volunteers, like ASHAs

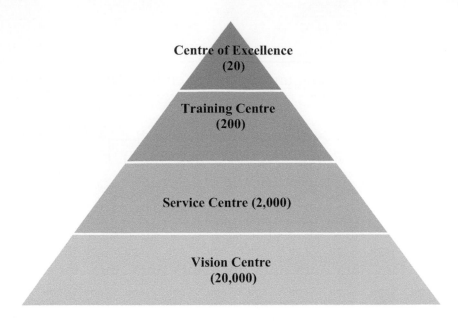

Figure 7.2 Vision 2020: The Right to Sight—pyramidal model of eye care in India.

Source: **Barrie Jones Lecture.**

7.7 VISION CENTRES

A vision centre is the first point of contact of the community with the eye care service provider. The eye care personnel at a vision centre are either a paramedical ophthalmic assistant or a vision technician, depending upon the model. There are various models of vision centres in India, but one thing is common, that it's a fixed facility, even if it is on wheels.

The centre is mostly meant for a population of 50,000. But again, this may vary across regions and across institutes. The centre is linked above to a base hospital, either government, charitable, or even private. The vision centre is connected to the community through some volunteers, like ASHAs in government set-up and vision guardians in private set-up.

Sustainability of vision centres is a challenge in non-government ones. To address this issue, the government of India, through NPCP&VI, is planning to increase the numbers of these vision centres in the public sector. It is planned to have it at the level of CHC initially, and later even at the PHC level. Sustainability in non-government sectors is ensured through revenue generation from spectacles and other services. Vision 2020: The Right to Sight, India, had planned for at least 20,000 vision centres by the year 2020. However, currently, there are around 4,000 VCs only.

There have been other models as well, like mobile centres which visit a set of same locations regularly for providing services to outreach difficult areas (5).

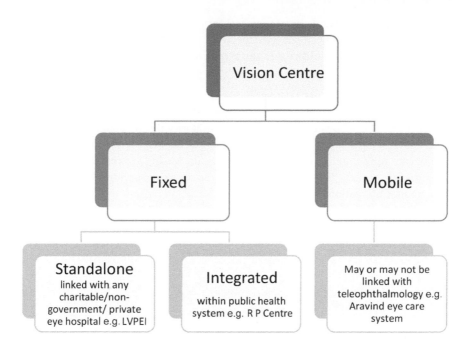

Figure 7.3 Various models of vision centres in India.

Sometimes, these centres may also be linked to higher centres through teleophthalmology to optimum care in real time.

7.8 HEALTH AND WELLNESS CENTRES

To provide a continuum of care to its citizens, the government of India initiated its flagship programme of Ayushman Bharat health and wellness centres (AB-HWCs) in 2018. Under this programme, comprehensive healthcare shall be provided at the level of sub-centres (now called HWCs) or at some places, even at the level of PHCs. The package of services would now be expanded from maternal and child health to include other important aspects of holistic care, like ophthalmic, ENT, dental, communicable, and non-communicable diseases. Target is to have at least 1.5 lakhs HWCs by the end of 2022 (6). The centre shall be manned by a mid-level health provider (MLHP)/community health officer (CHO) apart from the routine staff of sub-centre (7).

The list of eye care services that shall be made available at these HWCs are (8):

1. Screening for blindness and refractive errors through Snellen's chart.
2. Maintenance of blind register.
3. Generating awareness about common eye conditions, like conjunctivitis, refractive error, and cataract, and eye donation.

4. Providing first aid and prompt referral for ocular emergencies, like eye trauma, foreign body, burns, etc.
5. Identification of xerophthalmia and vitamin A prophylaxis.

7.9 COMMUNITY LEVEL

Eye problem is not considered a priority by majority of our people. This leads to sight-threatening scenario, when it could have been easily and completely managed if care were sought early. There is need for increasing awareness of the masses towards this aspect. This would improve their eye-care-seeking behaviour and hence better utilization of services.

It's imperative that there exist a smooth referral mechanism across the entire network of services. This link is complete only when the community is also looped in through their own community members. These link workers would increase the faith in services and provide complete information to the person seeking care.

Such workers are available in government set-up as ASHAs, accredited social health activists. ASHAs work in rural areas for every 1,000 population and in urban vulnerable areas for every 2,000 population. They are women with basic middle school education and belong to the same community. They provide incentive-based services. Mostly considered maternal and child workers, their role is also evolving, with a more comprehensive healthcare outlook of the government, which is the need of the hour.

Their counterparts in non-government set-up are the volunteers, like vision guardians, who provide exclusive services related to eye care and are linked and supported by standalone vision centres.

The activities related to eye care expected from ASHA workers are as follows (8):

1. Awareness generation on common eye disorders. Clarifying misconceptions related to eye care and eye disorders.
2. Facilitating people to receive eye care services and providing information about the same.
3. Ensuring vitamin A prophylaxis routinely for children under age 6 months to 5 years.
4. Referral and follow-up for availability of eye care services at referral centre.
5. Disbursing spectacles based on prescription, and ensuring regular use of spectacles.
6. Screening of visual impairment: less than 6/18 in any eye.
7. Symptomatic referral of patients with presbyopia, vision impairment, known diabetes, red eye, etc.
8. Maintaining a list of visually impaired and blind individuals in the community.

REFERENCES

1. Community Eye Health Journal . Perspectives on primary eye care [Internet]. [cited 2022 Jul 5]; Available from: www.cehjournal.org/article/perspectives-on-primary-eye-care/
2. World report on vision [Internet]. [cited 2022 Jul 5]; Available from: www.who.int/publications-detail-redirect/9789241516570
3. Definition of Primary Eye Care—2014—American Academy of Ophthalmology [Internet]. [cited 2022 Jul 5]; Available from: www.aao.org/clinical-statement/definition-of-primary-eye-care--policy-statement
4. Rao GN, Khanna RC, Athota SM, Rajshekar V, Rani PK. Integrated model of primary and secondary eye care for underserved rural areas: The L V Prasad Eye Institute experience. Indian J Ophthalmol 2012;60(5):396–400.
5. Misra V, Vashist P, Malhotra S, Gupta SK. Models for primary eye care services in India. Indian J Community Med Off Publ Indian Assoc Prev Soc Med 2015;40(2):79–84.
6. Bharat A. Health and Wellness Centres: 42. Available from: https://ab-hwc.nhp.gov.in/
7. Operational_Guidelines_For_CPHC.pdf [Internet]. [cited 2022 Jul 5]; Available from: www.nhm.gov.in/New_Updates_2018/NHM_Components/Health_System_Stregthening/Comprehensive_primary_health_care/letter/Operational_Guidelines_For_CPHC.pdf
8. Operational Guidelines for Eye Care at AB-HWC.pdf [Internet]. [cited 2022 Jul 5]; Available from: https://nhsrcindia.org/sites/default/files/2021-12/Operational%20Guidelines%20for%20Eye%20Care%20at%20AB-HWC.pdf

Health Promotion in Eye Care

SUMIT MALHOTRA

8.1 INTRODUCTION

Eye problems can occur from infancy to old age. Most of these are preventable and easily treatable if detected in the early stages. Moreover, disability arising due to these diseases seriously affects an individual's potential of leading a socioeconomically independent life (1, 2). Concerted efforts are imperative for promoting eye health at all levels of service provision, starting from community to tertiary healthcare levels. This chapter focuses on the theme of health promotion, its components and relevance to eye health.

8.2 HEALTH PROMOTION

Health promotion is the process of enabling people to increase control over and to improve their health.

The Ottawa Charter for Health Promotion was the first international conference on health promotion held from 17–21 November 1986. Health is a positive concept emphasizing social and personal resources as well as physical capacities. Therefore, health promotion is not just the responsibility of the health sector but goes beyond healthy lifestyles to well-being. Health promotion aims to achieve health equity by providing a solid foundation in a supportive environment, as well as access to information, life skills, and opportunities to make healthy choices. To account for differing social, cultural, and economic systems, health promotion strategies and programmes should be tailored to the local needs and capabilities of individual countries and regions (3).

In the Ottawa Conference's five key practical elements were included for health promotion. They were, namely:

1. Healthy public policy
2. Personal skills development
3. Community participation

    DOI: 10.1201/9781003291626-8

4. Supportive environments
5. Re-organization of health services

According to WHO, health promotion focuses on the following four aspects:

1. **Good governance.** This includes strengthening governance and policies that create an affordable and accessible healthcare system.
2. **Health literacy.** Improving health literacy in populations lays the groundwork for citizens to take an active role in improving their own health, participate successfully in community health action, and press governments to meet their responsibilities in addressing health and health equity.
3. **Healthy settings.** Healthy settings' key principles include community participation, partnership, empowerment, and equity, such as making sure there are safe places for people to exercise in urban areas.
4. **Social mobilization.** Bringing all societal and personal influences together to increase awareness and demand for healthcare, assist in the delivery of resources and services, and cultivate long-term individual and community involvement (4).

8.3 SUSTAINABLE DEVELOPMENT GOALS AND HEALTH PROMOTION

The 2030 agenda identifies 17 Sustainable Development Goals (SDGs) that aim to "ensure that all human beings can fulfil their potential in dignity and equality in a healthy environment." SDG 3 focuses on ensuring healthy lives and promoting well-being for all people at all ages. The 9th Global Conference (Shanghai 2016), titled "Promoting health in the Sustainable Development Goals: Health for all and all for health," highlighted the critical links between promoting health and the 2030 Agenda for Sustainable Development.

The Shanghai Conference identified the following key factors that will contribute to the success of health promotion for sustainable development:

- *Political commitment.* Many of the decisions needed to improve health require political will at the highest levels in order to promote health in all policies. Sustainable financial support for health promotion and public health is also critical.
- *Leadership for policy coherence.* Decisive leadership that champions the positive effects of good health on society as a whole makes a difference. Ministries of health, health agencies, and organizations play an important role in advocating for, facilitating, and mediating this leadership.
- *Capacity building to work in new ways.* Because of the rapidly changing environment and the increasing need for policy convergence, health promotion professionals must continuously build capacity. Working together to achieve the Sustainable Development Goals necessitates the development of

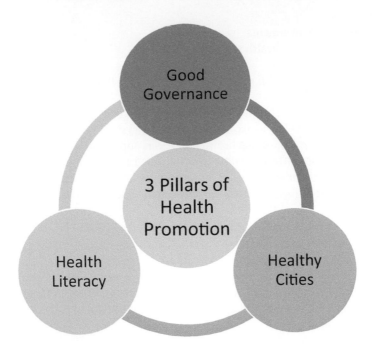

Figure 8.1 The three pillars of health promotion—good governance, healthy cities, and health literacy.

new skills for all actors involved in promoting health and well-being, from governments to civil society and the private sector.

- *Strong health promotion organizations.* These organizations are required for long-term health promotion action. Adaptable and integrative system capabilities are required as part of the overall public health system when implementing multisectoral and multidisciplinary approaches (5).

8.3.1 Health Promotion Strategies with Different Target Groups

1. **General Population**
   Health promotion activities can include population education on lifestyle modifications, such as healthy diet, regular exercise to prevent non-communicable disease, nutrition counselling in adolescents and women in reproductive age group, and awareness generation in school students.

2. **Population at Risk**
   This is for population groups that are at a high risk of developing a disease/disorder and exposed to risk factors. This includes targeted behavioural change strategies for population at risk and planning interventions to promote healthy behaviours and regular screening for NCDs.

3. **Individuals with Symptoms**

   Population here shows obvious signs of the disease condition. Home visits by frontline functionaries for early identification of symptoms, prompt referral, and follow-up of cases are useful in these types of cases.

4. **Population with Known Disorders**

   Few of the promotional interventions include individual and family counselling for treatment compliance and lifestyle modifications, disease-based patient support groups, and IEC activities using patient education leaflets, banners, posters, etc. (6).

8.3.2 Agents and Platforms for Health Promotion

1. **Frontline Workers**

   Frontline workers play a key role in the area of health promotion at community level. They raise public awareness of the various health and health-related services available to them and motivate them to use them. They also take the lead in the formation and operation of disease-specific patient support groups.

2. **Medical Officers**

   In addition to providing treatment, medical officers also plan and oversee individual and community-wide awareness and stigma-reduction activities.

3. **Vision Centres**

   A *vision centre* is a permanent eye care facility in the community which acts as the first point of interface of the population with comprehensive eye care services provided by an exclusive, skilled eye care worker. Its role includes but is not limited to early detection of eye problems, training of school teachers and preliminary screening by teachers, training and skill augmentation of other health/social development functionaries/volunteers, and conducting IEC activities (7).

4. **Village Committees, Women Collectives, and Self-Help Groups**

   Community-level forums promote intersectoral collaboration, local planning, and measures to solve issues of access and quality of care. They undertake large-scale community-level IEC activities planned in the form of campaigns, print material distribution, etc. and also inform people about various government programme and schemes.

5. **Patient Support Groups**

   The formation of patient support groups is facilitated by frontline workers to improve treatment compliance and engage not only those with the disease condition but also family members. Such groups would benefit patients and their families by providing mutual support, disease knowledge, increasing awareness about complications, combating discrimination and stigma associated with a specific disease, and enabling support for treatment continuation and changes in lifestyle behaviour (6).

6. **Health-Promoting Schools**

   A health-promoting school is one that constantly strengthens its capacity as a healthy setting for living, learning, and working. It promotes health and learning through all available means and engages health and education officials, teachers, teachers' unions, students, parents, healthcare providers, and community leaders in efforts to make the school a healthier environment. Strives to provide a healthy environment, school health education, and school health services, as well as school/community projects and outreach, health promotion programmes (8).

7. **Digital Platforms**

In today's day and age, when technology has become an integral part of our lives, digital platforms and social media play an important role in the area of health promotion. As a quick, interactive, and accessible medium, digital media has enormous potential to motivate and influence individuals, medical practitioners, and policymakers to improve health outcomes. Not only patients but also medical professionals and government agencies use various online platforms to communicate health-related information (9).

8.3.3 Digital Era and Health Promotion

In the digital age, a wide range of digitized health promotion strategies have emerged. Some of these practices are done voluntarily by people who want to improve their health and fitness, but many others are done for the benefit of organizations and agencies. The medium for these services is spread across the world in terms of applications ("apps"), websites, and platforms. These services provide easy access to medical and health information on the internet, new methods of monitoring, measuring, and visualizing the human body, as well as sharing personal information and experiences with others. As the most recent example, digital platforms were extensively used during the Covid-19 pandemic. Having said that, there are various challenges associated with digital health that include the exclusion of the poor and marginalized group and more of individual focus rather than community development and concerns about data privacy (9, 10).

8.3.4 Health Promotion and Eye Care

Strengthening general awareness and engaging and empowering people and communities are a key WHO recommendation in the World Report on Vision (2019). There is a compelling case for increasing health promotion and education in the field of eye care, given that the large majority of cases of vision impairment and blindness can be avoided through early detection and management. Poor eye health literacy can also limit medication adherence and routine eye examinations in people with chronic eye conditions. It is suggested that eye health promotion and education be provided at all levels of care, with a particular emphasis on integrating simple and effective education and counselling at the community and primary-care levels (11).

8.3.5 Elements of Health Promotion and Eye Care

1. *Healthy public policy.* Development of policies and programmes pertaining to eye care at various levels and understanding its importance in universal healthcare.

2. *Personal skills development.* The backbone of health promotion is health education, which encourages the adoption of eye-health-promoting behaviours and the utilization of eye care services. It also includes training of healthcare professional.
3. *Community participation.* Involving the community members at various levels of the programs gives them a sense of ownership with better compliance towards the programme.
4. *Supportive environments.* Having enabling and conducive environment is necessary. Like how accessibility to sanitation and safe, drinkable water is relevant in preventing trachoma.
5. *Re-organization of health services.* Improvements should address locally identified barriers, which might include quality of clinical care as well as all the other non-clinical aspects of care—for example, timing of clinics and operating sessions, ensuring men and women have separate waiting areas, providing culturally acceptable food and prayer areas, and ensuring a clean environment (12).

8.3.6 Health Promotion and Eye Care, India

The provision of health promotion and information at the community level is an essential component of the expanded range of services provided by the Comprehensive Primary Health Care. Health is influenced by a variety of social and environmental determinants, and actions to address these issues frequently fall outside the scope of health systems alone, necessitating intersectoral collaboration and public participation.

The eyes are an extremely delicate part of the body and hence need good care. This care begins at birth and continues throughout the life span. Health promotion activities at the Ayushman Bharat health and wellness centres (AB-HWC) will include regular awareness on care of the eye, identification of common eye-related symptoms, and the importance of seeking treatment early. For those suffering from blindness, health promotion activities will be centred on rehabilitation, regular check-ups, and reintegrating the person into the community.

Simple Eye Care Messages in Health Promotion

Infections of the eye spread very rapidly if proper care is not taken. The ways to maintain eye health are as follows:

1. Keep eyes clean by washing them with clean water. Washing eyes at bedtime is very good as it removes the dirt and dust collected throughout the day.
2. Do not work in poor light. Reading in poor light can strain eyes.
3. Always use a clean cloth to wipe eyes. Do not use saris, dhotis, or sleeves of clothes to wipe eyes. These may cause serious infection in

the eyes. Eye diseases such as conjunctivitis and trachoma spread by this way.

4. Each person should use a separate cloth, towel, or handkerchief for wiping eyes. If one eye is already infected, use a separate clean cloth for each eye.
5. Avoid the glare. Do not stare at the sun and other bright objects.
6. Never walk out in the sun without sunglasses.
7. Eat a diet rich in vitamin A and appropriate breastfeeding by mothers (colostrum is rich in vitamin A).
8. Do follow the 20–20–20 rule of eye care when using a computer/laptop, mobile phone, or watching television. Every 20 minutes, refocus your eyes for 20 seconds to an object located at least 20 feet away.
9. Report any eye infection to a health worker. Do not use home remedies for eye medication. Do not use medicines given by road-side medicine sellers. These may not help and may even cause blindness.
10. Eye drops and eye ointment only provided by a medical doctor should be used. Do not use any eye medicine without any medical prescription.
11. Educate community members to pay special attention in using eye drops. They might not make the difference between eye drops and ear drops and can put drops of the ear into their eyes.
12. Patients with eye infection should avoid going in swimming pools and visiting public places.

Source: Training Manual on Eye Care for Community Health Officer at Ayushman Bharat—Health and Wellness Centres.

Health Promotion at Community Level

Health promotion at the community level in India focuses on:

1. *Prevention.* Prevent eye problems in individuals by assisting them in adopting healthy eye care practices.
2. *Early detection and treatment.* If the disease is detected in initial stages and treated promptly, it can be controlled at an early stage.
3. *Education.* Spreading simple eye care messages to educate the community (13).

Services at Community Level

1. Awareness generation on common eye disorders and the need for early care-seeking through community-level meeting.
2. Clarifying misconceptions related to eye care and eye disorders, including discouraging the use of traditional eye medication or leftover eye drops.

Providing information about the availability of services related of eye treatment at different levels of healthcare.

3. Ensuring vitamin A prophylaxis routinely for children under age 6 months to 5 years.
4. Identifying/mobilizing patients with identified eye disease (of known diabetic, identified patients, or other disorders).
5. Referral and follow-up for availability of eye care services at referral centre.
6. Ensuring regular use of spectacles and follow-up biannually in children with refractive error.
7. Enabling the elderly and those with presbyopia to get free spectacles.
8. Encouraging eye examination for all children who were preterm (less than 32 weeks) or low birth weight (less than 2 kg) within 30 days.
9. Imparting health education for motivating people who are at risk of visual impairment.

Eye Health Promotional Messages for Mothers and Caregivers for Their Children

1. Clean their eyes immediately after birth. You can teach the mother/caregivers to provide eye care to the newborn, if required, by use of an eye ointment.
2. A baby with eye discharge needs treatment immediately; inform them to seek help from the nearest AB-HWC.
3. Make sure all mothers/caregivers report if their child is not looking at them or not looking straight after the age of 6 weeks. Mobilize the mother/caregivers for screening of children for eye care by Rashtriya Bal Swasthya Karyakram (RBSK) team.
4. Children should not play with or near sharp objects to avoid eye injuries.
5. Avoid applying "kajal" or "surma" in the eyes of the children.
6. Promote early and exclusive breastfeeding for the first six months of life.
7. Mothers and children should be fully immunized, including against rubella and measles.
8. Regular vitamin A supplementation of pre-school children from age of 9 months is important for good vision and healthy growth.
9. Children should eat foods rich in vitamin A to keep their eyes healthy.
10. Children should be made secure while travelling by taking all possible preventive measures to avoid eye injuries.

Source: Training Manual on Eye Care for Community Health Officer at Ayushman Bharat—Health and Wellness Centres.

8.4 ROLE OF FRONTLINE WORKERS IN EYE HEALTH PROMOTION

Frontline workers play an important role in conducting eye care promotion activities. It includes raising awareness for the prevention of eye disease (refractive error, cataract, trachoma, diabetic retinopathy, childhood blindness), maintaining personal hygiene and the environment, making lifestyle changes, and avoiding myths and misconceptions. They also contribute to raising awareness and mobilizing children for vitamin A prophylaxis and measles vaccination. Other responsibilities include using community-based platforms to educate people about eye care and changing the health-seeking behaviour of patients and caregivers through awareness and facilitation, as well as screening for blindness, visual impairment, and near vision (14).

8.4.1 Health Promotion Activities at Health and Wellness Centres

- Creating awareness about these contagious eye diseases through IEC to avoid the spread of these conditions, using appropriate measures.
- Awareness generation on common eye diseases and the need of seeking early eye care services whenever required.
- Awareness generation on eye donation.
- Educating the community regarding personal hygiene, facial cleanliness, and cleanliness of environment to prevent the spread of trachoma.
- Identifying vitamin A deficiency and Bitot's spot and assuring vitamin A prophylaxis.
- IEC activities, like avoiding touching the face and eyes during eye infections.

8.5 INTERSECTORAL COLLABORATION FOR HEALTH PROMOTION

Population health is determined not only by health sector activities but also by social and economic factors, and thus by policies and actions outside the purview of the health sector. As a result, it is critical for the health sector to collaborate with other sectors to raise awareness of the mutual benefits of working together for people-centred policies that promote health. This multisectoral collaboration can be attained by following a few strategies, like developing goals that align to the goals of different partners, inclusive and confident leadership, building trust between partners from the beginning, and considering the impact of political, economic, cultural, social, and organizational contexts. Regular monitoring and review help in emphasizing the importance of gauging how well the partnership is functioning at various stages of development, communicating successes, foreseeing upcoming issues, and learning from and responding to existing problems (15, 16).

REFERENCES

1. Vision impairment and blindness [Internet]. [cited 2022 Nov 21]. Available from: www.who.int/news-room/fact-sheets/detail/blindness-and-visual-impairment
2. Burton MJ, Ramke J, Marques AP, Bourne RRA, Congdon N, Jones I, et al. The Lancet Global Health Commission on Global Eye Health: vision beyond 2020. Lancet Glob Health [Internet]. 2021 Feb 16 [cited 2022 Nov 22];9(4):e489–551. Available from: www.ncbi.nlm.nih.gov/pmc/articles/PMC7966694/
3. Milestones in health promotion: statements from global conferences [Internet]. [cited 2022 Nov 22]. Available from: www.who.int/publications-detail-redirect/WHO-NMH-CHP-09.01
4. Health promotion [Internet]. [cited 2022 Nov 21]. Available from: www.who.int/health-topics/health-promotion
5. Promoting health in the SDGs: report on the 9th Global conference for health promotion, Shanghai, China, 21–24 November 2016: all for health, health for all [Internet]. [cited 2022 Nov 22]. Available from: www.who.int/publications-detail-redirect/promoting-health-in-the-sdgs
6. Operational_Guidelines_For_CPHC.pdf [Internet]. [cited 2022 Nov 23]. Available from: www.nhm.gov.in/New_Updates_2018/NHM_Components/Health_System_Stregthening/Comprehensive_primary_health_care/letter/Operational_Guidelines_For_CPHC.pdf
7. Vision-Centre-Manual-2012.pdf [Internet]. [cited 2022 Nov 24]. Available from: www.vision2020india.org/wp-content/uploads/2016/09/Vision-Centre-Manual-2012.pdf
8. Health promoting schools [Internet]. [cited 2022 Nov 24]. Available from: www.who.int/health-topics/health-promoting-schools
9. Kumari DS, Bharti A. Use of digital platforms for health promotion: a study of selected web portals. Eur J Mol Clin Med [Internet]. 2021 Feb 1 [cited 2022 Nov 24];7(7):4690–703. Available from: https://ejmcm.com/article_7306.html
10. Lupton D. Health promotion in the digital era: a critical commentary. Health Promot Int [Internet]. 2015 Mar 1 [cited 2022 Nov 24];30(1):174–83. Available from: https://doi.org/10.1093/heapro/dau091
11. World report on vision [Internet]. [cited 2022 Nov 21]. Available from: www.who.int/publications-detail-redirect/9789241516570
12. Community Eye Health Journal. Delivering eye health promotion: why and how [Internet]. [cited 2022 Nov 22]. Available from: www.cehjournal.org/article/delivering-eye-health-promotion-why-and-how/
13. Eye Care for FLW-Eye Health Promotion.pdf [Internet]. [cited 2022 Nov 23]. Available from: https://nhsrcindia.org/sites/default/files/2022-08/Eye%20Care%20for%20FLW-%20Eye%20Health%20Promotion.pdf
14. Operational_Guidelines_for_Primary_Eye_Care_at_HWCs.pdf [Internet]. [cited 2022 Nov 21]. Available from: https://ab-hwc.nhp.gov.in/download/document/Operational_Guidelines_for_Primary_Eye_Care_at_HWCs.pdf

15. Corbin JH, Jones J, Barry MM. What makes intersectoral partnerships for health promotion work? A review of the international literature. Health Promot Int [Internet]. 2018 Feb [cited 2022 Nov 24];33(1):4–26. Available from: www.ncbi.nlm.nih.gov/pmc/articles/PMC5914378/
16. Seventh Global Conference on Health Promotion, Nairobi, 26–30 October 2009 [Internet]. [cited 2022 Nov 24]. Available from: www.who.int/teams/health-promotion/enhanced-wellbeing/seventh-global-conference/partnerships

9

Ophthalmic Human Resources in the Country

SOUVIK MANNA, AMIT BHARDWAJ, PRAVEEN VASHIST

There are three pieces of information required before a healthcare plan can be developed:

- A description of how many people in the population of interest are affected, and how. This requires population-based surveys, epidemiological studies, and the use of routine data (census, government statistics, etc.) to collect information about prevalence, incidence, degree of severity, or the burden on the health system (number of people treated). This is called a needs assessment or epidemiological needs assessment.
- A description of the relevant resources available to the population of interest. The available resources, human, infrastructure, equipment, consumables, and financial, are identified using a variety of methods (information management systems, ad hoc surveys, interviews, etc.). It also includes an analysis of the utilization, effectiveness, and efficiency of the current services and the possible constraints. This is known as "situational analysis" or "corporate needs assessment."
- A description of what should be provided to deal with the condition in the population of interest. This is known as a "gap analysis" or "comparative needs assessment." It uses evidence of best practice, including published studies, as well as evidence from services to similar population within the same resource considerations, to establish what should be provided.

9.1 INDICATORS TO ASSESS HUMAN RESOURCE IN EYE CARE

9.1.1 District-Level Planning for HR

India is a union of 36 states/union territories comprising of 766 districts which serve as the most peripheral units of planning and programme implementation.

DOI: 10.1201/9781003291626-9

The population of the districts ranges from 8,000 in Upper Dibang Valley, Arunachal Pradesh, to 10 million in North 24 Parganas, West Bengal, with an average population of 2 million per district. The administration of the district is being maintained by district officials that include the following:

- *District magistrate (DM) or deputy commissioner or district collector.* An officer of the Indian Administrative Service (IAS), in charge of administration and revenue collection.
- *Superintendent of police (SP) or senior superintendent of police or deputy commissioner of police (DCP).* An officer belonging to the Indian Police Service (IPS), responsible for maintaining law and order.
- *Chief district health officer (CDHO).* An officer from the health cadre, responsible for public health and service delivery.

The World Health Organization (WHO) has also formulated a health systems framework that describes health systems in terms of six building blocks, acknowledging the health system strengthening agenda (1). These six building blocks are leadership/governance, healthcare financing, health workforce, medical products/technologies, information/research, and service delivery. The vital role of planning at the district level is evident from this classification. India has developed a strong service delivery mechanism for eye care since the inception of the National Program for Control of Blindness in 1976. The country presently has about 147,069 sub-health centres (SHCs) manned by two health workers for every 5,000 population in plains and 3,000 population in hilly/tribal/desert areas 23,391 primary health centres (PHCs) with a doctor and other paramedical staff for every 30,000 population in plains and 20,000 population in hilly/tribal/desert areas (2); 4,535 community health centres/first referral units (CHCs/FRUs) for every 120,000 population (3); and over 605 district and sub-district hospitals (DHs and SDHs) (4).

District is the most suitable administrative unit for decentralized planning below the state level, as it possesses the required heterogeneity and is small enough to undertake people in planning and implementation and to improve productivity; district planning is an important tool. The approach suggested for the preparation of the district plan is as follows:

- Preparation of district vision, block vision, and Gram Panchayat–level vision.
- Preparation of participatory plan, involving Gram Sabha from Gram Panchayats (GPs) to Zilla Parishad.
- Preparation of plans by urban local bodies (ULBs).
- Consolidation of plans prepared by local bodies by district planning committees.

Planning starts with the preparation of vision documents by local bodies (5).

Block-level planning. After finalizing the vision document for the district at the district level, the document shall be discussed at the block level, and a vision document for the block shall be prepared with some modifications based on the conditions of the block. The vision document for each block need not be completely different, because the conditions of some planning units at this level may be same.

Planning at the level of villages. At the third stage, the plan at the GPs/ULBs will be prepared. This will be prepared by the team with the help of community participation. They will first interact with the GP and prepare a vision on the lines of the district vision. Once the GP vision is approved, the team will conduct several focused group discussions (FGDs) to find out the potentials, needs, and constraints of the village economy in Gram Sabha. The felt needs of these communities and the support needed for improving their health conditions will be elicited. Once this exercise is completed, it will be discussed in the Gram Sabha. This approach will help study the situation thoroughly and prepare the plan. In particular, all the schemes will be examined thoroughly, with a view to understand their suitability to the community. This can be more easily ascertained from the beneficiaries/stakeholders. The plan should also take into account the long-term development perspective of the GP and also natural resource management (NRM) aspects.

District plan. The final stage is the preparation of the district plan. This will be finalized after the block plans are finalized in the same way as the block plan is finalized on the basis of the GP plans in the block. The schemes that will not figure in the block plans but are essential for the development of the district will be identified at this stage. Further, an attempt will have to be made to achieve functional and spatial integration and use the norms for the provision of social infrastructure.

Integration of entire local plan. For the realization of the district vision, district plans will need to put together resources channelized from all sources, including district segments to the state plan, centrally sponsored schemes (CSSs), grants-in-aids for specific purposes as provided by the NPCB&VI. Therefore, consolidation is a task that goes much beyond compilation and connotes a degree of value addition through integration of local plans. There are several aspects of integration of plans that have to be considered in the preparation of the draft development plan.

The different dimensions of integration have been discussed in the planning guidelines, as detailed in the following (6) (Figure 9.1).

9.1.2 Spatial Integration

This would mean integration of schemes that have an effect on one or more districts. Such kinds of eye care projects could be taken up with proportionate contributions from the districts concerned dovetailed into the funding available from above and entrusted to one local government for execution.

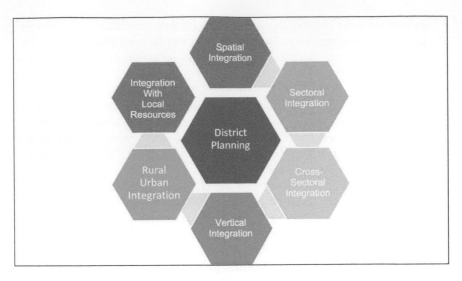

Figure 9.1 Different dimensions of integration in the preparation of district plans.

9.1.3 Sectoral Integration

This relates to the integration that takes place within a sector. For instance, an integrated approach to eye care would require the integration of several schemes relating to health, social justice, and education.

9.1.4 Cross-Sectoral Integration

To ensure maximum impact from different interventions, it is necessary to design approaches that draw resources from various schemes. For instance, a good approach to public health control of trachoma would require inputs from water and sanitation allocations and health programme allocations.

9.1.5 Vertical Integration

This is based on the precept that district and blocks ought to perform activities which have the advantages of scale and which cannot be done by the lower tiers of local government. This will require that blocks have a clear idea as to what the draft eye care plans contain; similarly, the district plans would need to consider the approved plans of village and blocks before finalizing theirs.

9.1.6 Integration of Resources

There are several schemes, both centrally sponsored and state sponsored, which districts can utilize, integrate into local plans, and to which they can contribute additional resources. There are several state plans, which, as implemented, can be strengthened by increased allocation from district funds. In some cases, a component having a complementary nature could be added to the state plan scheme. Similarly, CSSs should be integrated with district plans in the interest of efficient use of resources. There ought to be only one development plan for the district prepared through a common planning process and not a set of separate plans prepared in accordance with the guidelines of each programme. Thus, once priorities and works are identified and prioritized through a single planning process, components pertaining to a particular disease could be taken up through schemes, including CSSs, while still keeping within the guidelines of those schemes.

9.1.7 Integration with Local Resources

Planning can provide for local investments to be catalyzed through local resources or initiatives. By this, we do not mean that GPs ought to run industry locally but that it catalogues local skills and natural resource endowments and facilitate the development of business linkages. The public–private partnership model for spectacle distribution is a good example of this concept.

9.1.8 Rural–Urban Integration

Integration of urban–rural plans, which is particularly important in light of increasing urbanization, is an area where the district planning committee (DPC) could contribute a great deal. The DPC should work out mechanisms of joint programmes to be financed by state government institutions and joint contributions by urban and rural local bodies.

Vision 2020 has also recommended that each of their district-level Vision 2020 programmes should be for service units of about 1 million population (0.5–2 million) (7). The National Blindness and Visual Impairment Survey 2015–2019 (NBVI) was conducted in 31 districts of India, which provided district-level data on the magnitude of blindness and visual impairment. According to the survey, untreated cataract and cataract surgical complications cause 73.4% of the blindness in the country (8). The backlog of cataract blindness can only be cleared by providing quality surgeries at the district level. The other district-level indicators routinely reported are cataract surgical rate (CSR), which is defined as the total number of cataract surgeries per million population in a selected district per year. The current CSR (cataract surgical rate) of 5,000 is insufficient to make a dent on the problem of blindness. Moreover, bulk of the cataract surgeries are performed in metros and tier 1 and 2 cities, while the bulk of the cataract blindness exists in the rural hinterland, which has little access to quality eye care facilities (9).

The NBVI survey also draws attention to the glaring inequalities in eye healthcare system in India. Large parts of the country have little access to quality eye care even as super-specialty hospitals continue to crop up in big cities to cater to the country's rich. As far as human resources are concerned, there is wide variation in the doctor population ratio in various districts.

Recently, WHO has proposed two population-based indicators at district level, that is, effective cataract surgery coverage (eCSC) and effective refractive error coverage (eREC), that serve as ideal proxy indicators to not only track changes in the uptake and quality of eye care services at the global level but also contribute to monitoring progress towards universal health coverage (UHC) (10). The target has been set up as a 30 percentage points increase in eCSC and a 40 percentage points increase in eREC from the baseline to 2030 (10).

The government of India renamed the blindness programme as National Programme for Control of Blindness and Visual Impairment (NPCB&VI) in 2017, with a renewed focus on visual impairment and district-level planning. Various activities of the programme include the establishment of Regional Institutes of Ophthalmology (RIOs), upgradation of medical colleges and district hospitals (DHs) and block-level primary health centres, development of mobile units, and recruitment of required ophthalmic manpower in eye care units for the provision of various ophthalmic services. The programme aims to achieve its objectives by adopting decentralized implementation of the scheme through district health societies (DHS) of blindness. The pattern of assistance (2017–2020) for strengthening the districts involves:

- Assistance for the construction of dedicated eye units in DHs in north-eastern (NE) states and few other states as per need.
- Engagement of manpower, such as ophthalmic surgeons, eye donation counsellors, and data entry operators (DEOs), at district level on contractual basis to meet the shortage of manpower in the districts.
- Assistance for multipurpose district mobile ophthalmic units (MDMOUs) to improve coverage, comprising operating cost, including salary, maintenance, and POL (petroleum, oil, and lubricants), etc., @ Rs. 30 lakh per unit.
- Grant-in-aid for cataract operations in the government sector and NGO/private sector.

Incentives under the programme to community-level workers by the district health societies:

- ICDS functionaries, ASHA workers, and other voluntary groups, like mahila mandals/mahila arogya samitis (MAS), are eligible for a support of Rs. 350/operated case for identifying blind persons (blind registry), organizing and motivating identified persons, and transporting them to government/voluntary organizations fixed facilities for cataract surgeries, panchayats. If the patient is transported to the NGO facility for surgery, Rs. 350 shall be paid by the NGO out of Rs. 2,000 which it received as reimbursement for any free cataract surgery performed.
- Similarly, they are entitled to Rs. 350 for screening and distribution of free spectacles to school children and the elderly population.

Other grants-in-aids for strengthening the district involve:

- *Grant-in-aid for information, education, and communication (IEC) in the district.* The district-level activities include local IEC suitable to target population, use of folk methods and other indigenous means of communication, orientation of local leaders, etc.

- *Grant-in-aid for maintenance of ophthalmic equipment.* Maintenance of ophthalmic equipment @ Rs. 5 lakh per district to ensure longevity of costly ophthalmic equipment supplied under the programme.

Non-recurring grants-in-aids:

- *Strengthening of district hospitals/sub-district hospitals/PHCs (vision centres) in the government sector.* As per Indian Public Health Standards (IPHS) norms, the list of manpower and ophthalmic equipment for district hospitals/sub-district hospitals/vision centres has been provided with detailed guidelines.
- Grant-in-aid for eye donation centres amounts to up to Rs. 1 lakh per unit in public sector for strengthening/developing eye donation centres.

9.2 BASIC INFRASTRUCTURE AT DISTRICT LEVEL

Ideally, a district-level secondary eye care centre should be a 30- to 40-bed facility equipped to provide basic ophthalmic OPD services and surgical facilities up to cataract extraction with intraocular lens (IOL) implantation (11). Besides tackling cataract, this centre would also provide diagnostic, therapeutic, and surgical services for other common ocular conditions, like glaucoma, entropion, pterygium, etc., and would be suitably equipped to attend to all these problems efficiently. The support facilities in such a centre should include 24-hour power backup, round-the-clock water supply, hospital laundry and a hospital kitchen capable of catering to the patients and staff, an optical dispensing unit, and a pharmacy. The centre should also have spacious and comfortable accommodation for the resident team of surgeon(s), paramedics, and support service personnel besides (if feasible) a dedicated mobile unit vehicle for outreach activities.

9.2.1 Newer Initiatives for Cataract Elimination

The prevalence of blindness was 0.36% as per the National Blindness Survey from 2015–2019. In order to achieve the goal of 0.3% blindness, "Pradhan Mantri Motiyabind Abhiyaan" has been initiated successfully. The current level of blindness needs to be assessed using RAAB surveys at national level. In the population aged 50 years and above, the prevalence of blindness has remarkably declined over the past two decades from 5.3% in 2001 to 3.60% in 2007 to 1.99% in 2019 (8). A very ambitious programme of the MoHFW is the "PradhanMantri Motiyabind Abhiyan 2022–2025," with the target of completely covering the backlog of cataract surgeries leading to blindness and SVI among population aged 50 years and above. This translates to a target of 2.62 crore cataract surgeries in three years up to 2025. The achievement of these ambitious targets would require the implementation of all the components of the NPCB&VI in a mission mode. All the states/UTs are required to prepare a time-bound action plan comprising of the following components:

1. ***Districts as planning units.*** District-wise targets have been worked out as a proportion of the state/UT target, based on district population. Every district should aspire to achieve the "cataract blindness backlog–free" (CBBF) status by 2024–2025. District collectors should lead the campaigns in their respective districts. The district should also plan to become self-sufficient in surgical capacities in this period of three years so that CBBF status can also be achieved.

2. ***Primary screening of people for cataract.*** This may be organized through household surveys or through inclusion of this screening in the NCD screening using health and wellness centres (HWCs) as focal points. Focus of the primary screening should be to not miss out on any person aged 50 years or more.

3. ***Confirmatory screening and registration.*** Referral linkages may be set up for confirmatory screening of the people identified through primary screening, especially those aged 50 years or more, to shortlist people for cataract surgeries. A register of such identified people must be maintained.

4. ***Assessment of surgical capacities.*** A rapid assessment should be done to identify any gaps vis-à-vis the targets and the available surgical capacities. Capacities available in the private sector must also be taken into account. In order to leverage the private sector capacities, cataract surgery packages should be included in the PMJAY (Pradhan Mantri Jan Arogya Yojana), state insurance scheme packages, if not already included. Review of national insurance schemes reimbursement strategies for cataract surgery to minimize expenditure while maintaining quality services is needed. The resources available under the NPCB&VI may be utilized for this purpose in order to develop capacities up to the district hospital (DH) level.

5. ***Mapping of surgical safeguards and surgical capacities.*** Surgery schedules should be worked out, and districts with deficit in capacities must be suitably mapped with districts having surplus capacities. Review of cataract surgical services performance and outcomes, including patient perception of services, is also important.

6. ***Training.*** Training needs may be identified, and arrangements for training should be planned for (a) primary screening, (b) confirmatory screening, (c) cataract surgical capacities, (d) infection prevention protocols, and (e) follow-up care.

7. ***Logistics for essential supplies.*** Timely arrangement of essential supplies, such as lenses, spectacles, sutures, and other consumables, will be critical for the successful implementation of the programme. They must be planned and implemented in a time-bound manner to avoid any delays.

The key component here is the bridging strategy linking the communities in need to the hospital clinical services—concentrating on what can be achieved, with a particular disease intervention in an accessible part of the district, rather than setting objectives that will require substantial additional resources (12). The WHO estimates that an ophthalmologist can be expected to perform 1,000–2,000 cataract operations per year, if they are well supported and patients present for surgery (13). Often, the clinicians are concentrated in larger urban centres, with rural populations relatively underserved (14).

9.3 NEED FOR EYE CARE IN A MILLION POPULATION IN INDIA

India has the largest magnitude of blindness and visual impairment in the world, in numbers disproportionate to its proportion of global populations. The age-standardized proportion of people who need refractive services, annual eye examinations, cataract surgical services, and low vision services is 55.6%, 40.0%, 13.4%, and 0.8%, respectively, in Indians (15). The Vision 2020 approach proposes that activities should be planned and implemented for a defined population and geographical coverage and promotes the concept of a manageable unit of a population of 500,000 to 1 million, termed a Vision 2020 delivery unit (16). Recommendations on targets for services and resources required have been made as unit ratios of the delivery unit, for example, two to four ophthalmologists, four to ten ophthalmic nurses per delivery unit. This implies that there is a team responsible for the eye health of the population of a Vision 2020 delivery unit. So if projected to a million population, the number of Indians in need are (Table 9.1):

The aspirational districts programme of the government of India also provides special emphasis on the districts lagging behind in terms of eye care facilities. District health societies (DHSs) under the National Health Mission (NHM) have been created for decentralized programme management throughout the country under the chairmanship of the district collector/deputy commissioner (17). Centrally collected data on eye care in the country is collected at the district level through DHS and disaggregated by age and gender. However, progress to reduce inequity in eye care services coverage is not reviewed regularly.

There is an urgent need to work towards balancing the inequality in terms of health workforce and services to ensure a more equitable distribution of health resources. District-level planning plays a central role in shifting the onus of planning from the central to the peripheral levels. Further, the CNAA (community needs assessment approach) should be employed, in which plans regarding health

Table 9.1 Number of Indians in Need of Various Eye Care Services

Services	Need (Per Million)	Daily OPD Needed	OPD/Mobile Van/Day
Refractive services	5,56,000	2,000	600
Annual eye examination services	4,00,000	1,600	500
Cataract surgical services	1,34,000	500	150
Low-vision services	80,000	300	100

services are to be formulated in consultation with the community at the grassroots level and expected to lead to improvement in quality of services and client satisfaction matching with ground situation requirements (18).

REFERENCES

1. Everybody's business—strengthening health systems to improve health outcomes: WHO's framework for action [Internet]. [cited 2022 Jul 7]. Available from: https://apps.who.int/iris/handle/10665/43918
2. Sriram S. Availability of infrastructure and manpower for primary health centers in a district in Andhra Pradesh, India. J Fam Med Prim Care. 2018;7(6):1256–62.
3. Directorate General of Health Services. Indian Public Health Standards (IPHS) Guidelines for Community Health Centres. Rural Health Statistics Bulletin. 2012. pp. 1–79.
4. Directorate General of Health Services. Indian Public Health Standards (IPHS) Guidelines for District Hospitals. Rural Health Statistics Bulletin. 2012. pp. 1–110.
5. Planning Commission of India. Manual for Integrated District Planning. Planning Commision of India. 2008. pp. 1–157.
6. Kerala State Planning Board [Internet]. [cited 2022 Sep 30]. Available from: https://spb.kerala.gov.in/en/decentralised-planning-division
7. Cook B, Babar Q. VISION 2020 at the district level. Community Eye Health J. 2005;18. pp. 85–89.
8. Vashist P, Senjam SS, Gupta V, Gupta N, Shamanna BR, Wadhwani M, Shukla P, Manna S, Yadav S, Bharadwaj A. Blindness and visual impairment and their causes in India: results of a nationally representative survey. PLoS One. 2022 Jul;17(7):e0271736.
9. Keel S, Müller A, Block S, Bourne R, Burton MJ, Chatterji S, et al. Keeping an eye on eye care: monitoring progress towards effective coverage. Lancet Glob Heal [Internet]. 2021 Oct 1 [cited 2022 Jul 14];9(10):e1460–4. Available from: https://pubmed.ncbi.nlm.nih.gov/34237266/
10. Ramke J, Gilbert CE, Lee AC, Ackland P, Limburg H, Foster A. Effective cataract surgical coverage: an indicator for measuring quality-of-care in the context of Universal Health Coverage. PLoS One. 2017;12(3):1–13.
11. Goel H. District level eye care delivery system. Community Eye Heal [Internet]. 2005;18(54):S61–64. Available from: http://hy8fy9jj4b.search. serialssolutions.com.libraryproxy.griffith.edu.au/?ctx_ver=Z39.88-2004&ctx_enc=info%3Aofi%2Fenc%3AUTF-8&rfr_id=info%3Asid%2Fsummon.seri-alssolutions.com&rft_val_fmt=info%3Aofi%2Ffmt%3Akev%3Amtx%3Ajourn al&rft.genre=article&rft.atitl
12. VISION 2020 at the district level. Community Eye Health. 2005 Jun;18(54):85–9. PMID: 17491756; PMCID: PMC1705676.
13. World Health Organization. Elimination of avoidable blindness. World Heal Organ. 2003;2003–6.

14. Katibeh M, Blanchet K, Akbarian S, Hosseini S, Ahmadieh H, Burton M. Planning eye health services in Varamin district, Iran: a cross-sectional study. BMC Health Serv Res. 2015 Apr 3;15:140.
15. Zheng Y, Cheng CY, Lamoureux EL, Chiang PPC, Anuar AR, Wang JJ, et al. How much eye care services do Asian populations need projection from the Singapore epidemiology of eye disease (SEED) study. Investig Ophthalmol Vis Sci. 2013;54(3):2171–7.
16. Faal H. Reaching into the district: strengthening the eye care team. Community eye Heal. 2004 Oct;17(51):36–7.
17. Jose R, Bachani D. World bank-assisted cataract blindness control project. Indian J Ophthalmol. 1995 Jan 1;43(1):35–43.
18. MedCosmos PSM: CNAA-community needs assessment approach [Internet]. [cited 2022 Sep 30]. Available from: http://medcosmospsm.blogspot.com/2008/09/cnaa-community-needs-assessment.html

10

Introduction to Health Economics

B. R. SHAMANNA, SUNNY MANNAVA

10.1 INTRODUCTION TO HEALTH ECONOMICS

Economics is a discipline which is both an art and a science. It is a "science of scarcity" and an "art of resource" allocation. Health economics is a field of economics that focuses on the "analysis and understanding of efficiency, effectiveness, values and behaviours involved in the production and consumption of health and healthcare." Health economists are interested in the efficient design of healthcare systems (including social security systems), the economic evaluation of health technologies, health-related behaviours, and the impacts of incentives, financial and otherwise, to modify these behaviours (1). The simple explanation is that it is a discipline that determines the price and the quantity of limited financial and non-financial resources devoted to the care of the sick and promotion of health. It is also about applying the principles of economics to the field of health and healthcare.

10.2 BASIC NOTIONS OF HEALTH ECONOMICS

Health economics outlines a few notions which are like its principles that guide its utility and use. These are:

- Human wants are unlimited, but resources are limited and finite.
- Economics is as much about benefits as it is about costs.
- Costs and consequences are not restricted to the hospital, or even to the health sector.
- Choices in healthcare inescapably involve value judgments.
- Many of the simple rules of market operation do not apply in the case of healthcare.
- Consideration of costs is not necessarily unethical.

DOI: 10.1201/9781003291626-10

- Most choices in healthcare relate to changes in the level or extent of a given activity; the relevant evaluation concerns these marginal changes and not the total activity.
- The provision of healthcare is but one way of improving the health of the population.
- As a community, we prefer to postpone costs and to bring forward benefits.
- Equity in healthcare may be desirable, but reducing inequalities usually comes at a price.

10.3 THE CONCEPT OF OPPORTUNITY COST

The whole discipline of health economics is dependent on the concept of "opportunity cost." The decision to use a resource (people, time, facility, equipment, etc.) in one area always involves a cost. That is, the opportunity to use it to produce benefits in another area must be foregone. This is the understanding of opportunity cost. For example, resources for HIV control programmes, if needed to be allocated, have to be at the cost of another programme, like a malaria control programme. Also, a curative programme in the same discipline, like a bypass heart surgery, may be at the cost of a preventive cardiology health education initiative. This is called an "opportunity" cost.

10.4 THE PRINCIPLE OF ALLOCATIVE EFFICIENCY

In the discipline of economics, there are two principles of economic efficiency, namely:

- *Productive/technical/operational efficiency.* Achieving maximum output at a given cost or a given output at minimum cost. It is about doing things right (efficiency) (2, 3).
- *Allocative efficiency.* Situation where no reallocation can make one individual better off without making at least one worse off. It is about doing the right things (effectiveness) to maximize the health of the society (2, 4).

Health economics, unlike market economics, is skewed more towards allocation of available scarce resources than productive or technical efficiency. The felt need and consumer preference within a societal context decide the allocation of limited resources in health economics.

10.5 USES OF HEALTH ECONOMICS

Broadly, health economics has its utility in:

- Allocation of resources between various health-promoting activities.
- Quantity of resources used in health delivery.

- Organization and funding of health institutions.
- Efficiency of how resources are allocated and used for health issues.
- Allocation to preventive, curative, and rehabilitative health services and its effects on society.

Health economics consciously looks at resource allocation and tries to ensure equity, effectiveness, efficiency, and excellence/quality in service care delivery. It is also very pertinent that economics needs to be distinguished from accountancy and, especially, health economics, as there is an emotional connect with the logical aspect of allocating resources. The application of economics to healthcare requires quantification, prediction, and evaluation as the situation warrants when resources are being invested.

The discipline of health economics also looks at microeconomics, which focuses on the actions of individual agents within the economy, like households, workers, and businesses. At a larger level, it also looks at macroeconomics, which looks at the economy as a whole. Here, it focuses on broad issues, such as growth of production, the number of unemployed people, the inflationary increase in prices, government deficits, and levels of exports and imports. Microeconomics and macroeconomics are not separate subjects but, rather, complementary perspectives on the overall subject of the economy. Economists use the scientific method to generalize and derive abstractions to develop theories. This is called theoretical economics. These theories are then applied to fix problems or meet economic goals. This is called policy economics. Health economics looks at policy economics in more detail as it is about allocative efficiency.

10.6 EQUITY, DEMAND, SUPPLY, AND PRICE EQUILIBRIUM

10.6.1 Equity

Equity in healthcare refers to the distribution of resources fairly across individuals (4). There are two concepts of equity: *horizontal equity* refers to "equal treatment of equals" or "equal access for equal need" (5), and *vertical equity* refers to "unequal but equitable treatment of unequals" (6, 7). This is harder to achieve because of resource scarcity, as a programme which is targeted to eliminate blindness due to cataract may leave out children with blindness, leaving an inequitable health outcome for the society.

10.6.2 Demand

It is the choice of the consumer over the consumption of specific goods. When the price goes up, the quantity demanded for a good goes down, with all else being equal (8). Demand for healthcare is different from other types of demands, as demand for healthcare is a "derived" demand, wherein the demand is a fundamental demand for good health (9).

10.6.3 Price Elasticity of Demand

It measures the responsiveness of quantity demanded for a good or service to change in its own price (8). The percentage change in quantity demanded divided by the associated percentage change in price:

$$\frac{\left(D_2 - D_1\right)}{D_1} \Big/ \frac{\left(P_2 - P_1\right)}{P_1}$$

10.7 SUPPLY

"It is the willingness and the ability to sell a good over each and various prices over a given time period" (8). Supply varies over time and across states and districts due to scarce resources and factors such as availability of healthcare professionals, budget size, production technology, logistics, etc. (9).

10.7.1 Price Elasticity of Supply

It measures the responsiveness of the quantity supplied of a good or service to change in its own price (8). The percentage change in quantity supplied of a good or service divided by the percentage change in the good's own price:

$$\frac{\left(S_2 - S_1\right)}{S_1} \Big/ \frac{\left(P_2 - P_1\right)}{P_1}$$

10.7.2 Price Equilibrium

It is a situation where, for a given price, the quantity demanded is equal to the quantity supplied (8). Sometimes the price of equilibrium may be high to keep the supply and demand constant.

10.7.3 Externality

An *externality* is a cost or a benefit associated with one person's activity that impacts others who did not choose to incur that cost or benefit (10). An externality can be both positive or negative and can stem from either the production or consumption of a good or service. The costs and benefits can be both private, to an individual or an organization, or social, meaning, it can affect society as a whole.

An externality usually does not affect the entity that causes the externality. A positive externality occurs where social benefit of consumption of good exceeds private benefit (e.g. herd immunity). In a negative externality, the social cost of consumption of good exceeds private cost (e.g. pollution). Health economics requires decisions that manage the interaction between the mission of the programme and the externalities involved.

10.8 THE EPIDEMIOLOGICAL BASIS OF HEALTH ECONOMICS (11)

Health economics is very dependent on basic epidemiological concepts, that is, the efficacy and effectiveness criteria. Further, prior to carrying out any economic evaluation, questions need to be posed and answered, namely, Can it work? Does it do more good than harm? What about compliance? Does it work under ordinary practice conditions? These are aspects that cement the connect between epidemiology and health economics.

10.9 ECONOMIC EVALUATION IN (EYE) HEALTHCARE

10.9.1 Overview

Let us imagine you are a key stakeholder in the decision-making process of allocating budget towards a programme aimed at reducing the prevalence of blindness in an area. Two programmes are proposed; one aims to conduct recurrent screening programmes in the area, and the other aims to establish a vision centre (Figure 10.1). Due to resource scarcity, only one of the two programmes can get budgetary allocation. How do you decide which programme to support? A lot of factors, including costs and benefits, are considered to arrive at a decision to choose one programme over another, and more precisely, this process is called an economic evaluation (11). *Economic evaluation* is "the comparative analysis where it compares two options in-terms their costs and consequences" (12). Economic evaluation answers resource utilization, impact of a programme, loss, expenditure, budget, stakeholder participation, consequences, decision on alternative choices (9, 12). The tasks of economic evaluations are to identify, quantify, value, and compare the costs and the consequences.

Valuation of costs are important to undertake the economic evaluation. Costs denote the consumption of resources to be converted through a process to achieve the consequences, which are then compared among two or more alternatives before a choice is made in the economic evaluation. The economic

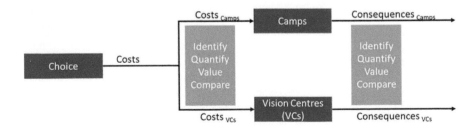

Figure 10.1 Understanding economic evaluation in eye healthcare—comparative analysis.

Source: **Drummond et al. (2015) (12).**

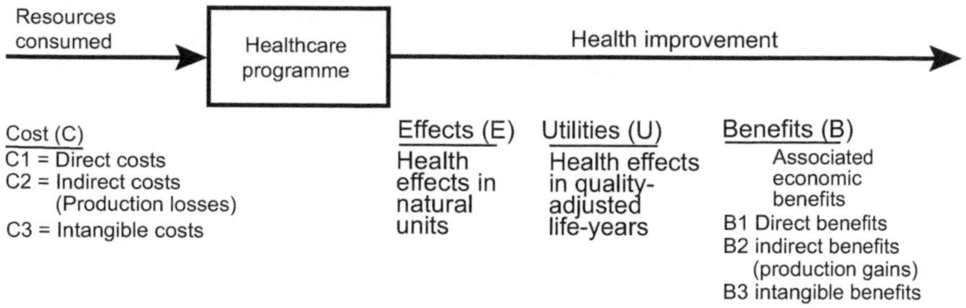

Figure 10.2 Understanding costs and consequences involved in full economic evaluation.

Source: **Figure adapted from the textbook of Mike Drummond (13).**

evaluation can be full or a partial. A full economic evaluation requires that costs, consequences of two or more alternatives, are compared before a choice is made using an agreed criterion. Any other comparison will fall into a partial economic evaluation analysis.

Costs are classified as direct, indirect, and intangible costs; fixed and variable costs; capital and recurrent costs; marginal and incremental costs; as well as transfer payments, while undertaking the valuation of the inputs in an economic evaluation.

10.10 CRITERIA AND PERSPECTIVES IN A HEALTH ECONOMIC EVALUATION

The choice of the most economically efficient intervention depends on the criteria that may be useful in deciding among different uses for limited resources. These criteria, most often than not, are evidence-based and explicit. There are, at times, criteria that may be adopted which can only be implicit (Covid-19 lockdown). Economic analysis seeks to identify one set of criteria that may be useful in deciding among different uses for limited resources.

The perspectives in an economic evaluation depend on from whose viewpoint the evaluation is carried out. These can be people (society), patient, provider, or payer (insurance) perspective, and accordingly, the comparison and choice are carried out. The broadest perspective is peoples' or societal, which reflects a full range of social opportunity costs associated with different interventions.

There are three full commonly used types of economic evaluations.

10.11 STAGES/PHASES OF ECONOMIC EVALUATION (9)

- *Defining/framing the evaluation.* It is very important to clearly define why you need to carry out the economic evaluation, purpose of the evaluation,

Table 10.1 Types of Economic Evaluations

Type of Analysis	Measurement/ Valuation of Costs in Both Alternatives	Identification of Consequences	Measurement/ Valuation of Consequences
Cost-effectiveness analysis	Monetary units	Single effect of interest common to both alternatives but achieved to different degrees	Natural units (e.g. life-years gained, disability days saved, gain in visual acuity, etc.) Incremental cost-effectiveness ratio (ICER); average cost-effectiveness ratio (ACER)
Cost–utility analysis	Monetary units	Single or multiple effects, not necessarily common to both alternatives	Healthy years, typically measured as quality-adjusted life-years (QALY) or disability-adjusted life-year (DALY)
Cost–benefit analysis	Monetary units	Single or multiple effects, not necessarily common to both alternatives	Monetary units; net present value (NPV); benefit–cost ratio (BCR)

Source: Drummond et al. (2015) (12).

who are the stakeholders (in this case, the beneficiaries, programme team, funding source, community), audience (funding agency, government, other partners), time frame (time course for camps and/or vision centre and their start-up[1] and maintenance costs,[2] along with discounting), perspectives (societal perspective and health system perspective), interventions for comparison.

- *Identifying, quantifying, and valuing the resources needed.* This is not a simple and easy exercise, as it involves inputs from a lot of areas. Cost of resources may be majorly classified as:
  1. **Direct costs (direct medical and direct non-medical).** Direct medical costs are those which are spent on implementation and continuation of the health service/intervention (on community screening or vision centre). Direct non-medical costs are those which are spent on non-healthcare, such as transport to and from community or vision centre.
  2. **Indirect costs.** Costs incurred by the patient, such as the patient's and family member or caregiver's time going to the hospital. Measured in terms of the foregone wages or earnings.
  3. **Intangible costs.** These are the costs which cannot be measured monetarily, such as emotions, pain, and suffering of the patient due to the intervention. They may not be measured, but they have to be considered during decision-making as they have a huge bearing on the consequence, as it would influence the community's acceptance of the intervention.
- *Identifying, quantifying, and valuing the health consequences.* Measuring health consequence depends on the type of disease, intervention, and outcome. The consequences may be tangible in most cases or intangible in some cases. Tangible consequences for interventions, such as community screening or vision centre, could be an improvement in the visual acuity of the patients in the area of intervention, improvement in the quality of life, increased labour participation. The intangible consequence could be an adverse effect due to over-correction of myopia at camp or vision centre. An individual's preference for a health state is called "utility weight" or "utility" (14). Utility weights are used to generate DALYs and QALYs, which are used in cost–utility analyses (CUAs). A combination of length and quality of life is QALY. Having more QALYs means that the individual will live longer and healthier. Considering the utility value for blindness as 0.57 (15), the QALY for an individual living with blindness for 10 years would be 5.7 versus an individual treated for blindness, whose QALY would be 10, indicating that there is 4.3 QALY gain due to intervention. Similarly, DALYs are a measure of healthy time lost due to a disease. Healthcare programs aim to reduce DALYs (16).
- *Presenting and interpreting the evidence for decision-making.* Depending on the type of analysis, one must compare the results of economic analysis for both the interventions.

For cost–benefit analyses (CBAs), compare NPV or BCR:
Net Present Value (NPV)

$$NPV = \sum_{t=0}^{n} \frac{\left(Benefits - Costs\right)_t}{\left(I + r\right)^t}$$

where:

r = discount rate
t = year
n = analytic horizon (in years)

A positive and higher NPV of an intervention would indicate that the intervention is beneficial to the society as the benefits outweigh the costs.
Benefit–Cost Ratio (BCR)

$$BCR = \frac{PV_{Benefits}}{PV_{Costs}}$$

Where:

$PV_{Benefits}$ = present value of benefits
PV_{Costs} = present value of costs
BCR greater than 1 is beneficial.

For cost-effectiveness analyses (CEAs), compare ICER or ACER:
Incremental Cost-Effectiveness Ratio (ICER)

$$ICER = \frac{Total\,Costs_{Intervention\,A} - Total\,Costs_{Intervention\,B}}{Total\,Effects_{Intervention\,A} - Total\,Effects_{Intervention\,B}}$$

ICER is used to compare two alternative interventions. Intervention with a lower ICER is preferred.
Average Cost-Effectiveness Ratio (ACER)

$$ACER = \frac{Total\,Costs_{Intervention\,A}}{Total\,Effects_{Intervention\,A}}$$

ACER is for singe intervention, which is compared against no intervention.

For cost–utility analyses (CUAs), compare QALY or DALY: Cost per QALY gained or DALY averted is used to compare interventions.

10.12 SENSITIVITY ANALYSIS

Sensitivity analysis needs to be undertaken on those estimates, which have a higher degree of variability, as costs are subject to uncertainty. Discounting is another aspect that is used in an economic evaluation to adjust for differential timing of costs and consequences and is very important to provide a level playing field during the comparison of the interventions.

10.13 USES OF AN ECONOMIC EVALUATION

The economic evaluations are useful for:

- *Healthcare planning.* Which programme should receive more resources—deafness or AIDS?
- *Third-party payers.* What insurance premiums? Service package?
- *Hospital administrators.* Investment? Equipment and its returns?
- *Physicians.* Plan and provide services—cost of services? Hearing aids vs. cochlear implant?
- *End users.* Patients for seeking and utilizing treatment.

10.14 THE ECONOMIC BURDEN OF BLINDNESS

10.14.1 Background

Blindness leads to greater individual and societal losses. Most studies estimate the economic burden of blindness in terms of loss of productivity or willingness to pay. The oldest and the most common method to express the economic burden of a disease or illness, including blindness, is the cost of illness method (17, 18). Cost of illness studies evaluate the productivity losses and utilization of healthcare resources due to an illness and assume that there will be economic benefits if a health intervention addresses the underlying disease (19). Various studies have used several different methods to estimate cost of blindness (20–25) across the world. Most of the literature evidence surrounding cost of illness studies contains a lot of heterogeneity in terms of the methodology used globally (23, 26). The estimates are based mainly on the prevalence or incidence of disease; direct costs, which include actual expenses incurred, including medical, non-medical, and other costs; indirect costs, which include the foregone income and loss of productivity due to absenteeism by the patient and caregiver; and intangible costs, such as loss of quality of life, expressed as DALYs (20, 27).

10.14.2 Current Estimates of the Economic Burden of Blindness

Globally, there are an estimated 43 million people blind and 553 million people visually impaired, classified as per the WHO definition of blindness and visual impairment (28, 29). As per a systematic review done in the year 2013, the cost of blindness per blind individual per year in the world is US$ PPP 14,882–24,180 (21). Potential loss of productivity due to blindness in the world is estimated to be US$ PPP 43.6 billion (23). The economic burden is highest in East and South Asia. As per Mannava et al. (2022), the economic burden of blindness in India is US$ PPP 11 billion (INR 845 billion) in 2020, the direct loss is US$ PPP 10 billion (INR 768 billion), the indirect loss is US$ PPP 1.9 billion (INR 144 billion), and the cumulative loss due to blindness over the lifespan of the blind is INR 22,565 billion (24). This study used direct costs due to blindness, indirect costs due to blindness, and considered the lowered contribution of the blind persons towards the economy of India (24). This study used prevalence estimates and per capita income and the assumption that 60% of the blind adults could have contributed to the labour force if they were not blind, in order to calculate the economic burden of blindness (24). Another study done by B. Wong et al. (2021) in India found that the economic burden of blindness in India is US$ PPP 2.8 billion (INR 214 billion); there were not cumulative loss estimates reported in this study (25). This study expressed the economic burden of blindness in India by considering parameters such as prevalence, loss of employment, productivity loss, and caregiver costs (25). Although both the studies considered the same prevalence of blindness, the difference in the numbers is mainly due to the different estimations of the prevalence denominator due to the lack of current population data, different sources considered for labour force participation, and differences in loss of employment estimates.

Although there is a lot of debate about cost-of-illness studies and their lack of consideration of individual and societal perspectives of the disease (19, 27), they still remain the most common tool to estimate the economic burden of blindness. They are used as important policy drivers enabling advocacy and recommend budgetary allocations. Cost of illness studies enable researchers to undertake economic burden of disease studies on a large population setting and hence are used by the World Health Organization (WHO) and the World Bank. However, they are not useful in understanding the impact of healthcare programmes targeted towards the reduction in the prevalence of blindness, and hence, other approaches, such as cost-effectiveness and cost–utility analysis, need to be undertaken to carry out economic evaluations of such programmes.

10.14.3 Critical Appraisal of Economics Evaluation Article or a Publication (11)

A guidance, as follows, is provided as a broad framework for learners to critically appraise and understand a publication which is in the realm of an article on economic evaluation. These are:

- What is the research question asked or posed? Is it in an answerable form?
- Was there epidemiological evidence that showed that the considered interventions were effective before performing an economic evaluation?
- Has there been a complete description of the interventions considered for economic evaluation?
- What is the type of economic evaluation that has been performed?
- Whose perspective has been considered?

- Has costs and consequences been valued/measured? And how?
- What costs are considered, and how have they been compared?
- What consequences have been considered, and how have they been compared?
- Were costs and consequences adjusted for differential timing (discounting)?
- Have they performed any analysis for uncertainty (sensitivity analysis)?
- Is there any incremental analysis performed?
- Has there been a choice made or recommended based on the analysis performed and why?
- Did they mention limitations in the approach they used?
- Any other information?

10.15 SUMMARY

Economic evaluations help us decide on which intervention to choose where resources are scarce and need to be allocated efficiently. Although the benefits may be higher, some interventions may be rejected if the upfront costs are higher than the available budget. Tools such as the World Health Organization Choosing Interventions That Are Cost-Effective (WHO CHOICE) (30) may help in generalized quantitative assessment of large programmes and health systems. The Consolidated Health Economic Evaluation Reporting Standards 2022 (CHEERS 2022) (31) needs to be used in every economic evaluation where two alternatives are compared. Further research is needed in developing a database of utility values for various health outcomes in Indian scenario which would help in carrying out economic analyses. It has to be understood that economic evaluation is a tool that can be used to prioritize and allocate scarce resources. Ultimately, it needs to be used along with societal needs and budgetary allocations to prioritize allocation of scarce resources.

NOTES

1 *Start-up costs* are those needed to set up the camp or vision centre.
2 *Maintenance costs* are those that are needed to keep the programme running.

REFERENCES

1. Health Economics—YHEC—York Health Economics Consortium [Internet]. [cited 2022 Oct 5]. Available from: https://yhec.co.uk/glossary/health-economics/
2. Health Systems Governance and Financing [Internet]. [cited 2022 Oct 5]. Available from: www.who.int/teams/health-systems-governance-and-financing/economic-analysis/costing-and-technical-efficiency/technical-efficiency
3. Palmer S, Torgerson DJ. Economics notes: Definitions of efficiency. Br Med J [Internet]. 1999 Apr 4 [cited 2022 Oct 5];318(7191):1136. Available from: / pmc/articles/PMC1115526/

4. Equity—YHEC—York Health Economics Consortium [Internet]. [cited 2022 Oct 5]. Available from: https://yhec.co.uk/glossary/equity/

5. Mooney GH. Economics, medicine and health care. Pearson Education; 2003.

6. Shiell A, Donaldson C, Mitton C, Currie G. Health economic evaluation. J Epidemiol Community Heal [Internet]. 2002 Feb 1 [cited 2022 Oct 5];56(2):85–8. Available from: https://jech.bmj.com/content/56/2/85

7. Mooney G. And now for vertical equity? Some concerns arising from aboriginal health in Australia. Health Econ [Internet]. 1996 [cited 2022 Oct 5];5(2):99–103. Available from: https://onlinelibrary.wiley.com/doi/epdf/10.1002/%28SICI%291099-1050%28199603%295%3A2%3C99%3A%3AAID-HEC193%3E3.0.CO%3B2-N

8. Guinness L, Wiseman V. Introduction to health economics. 2nd ed. Guinness L, Wiseman V, editors. McGraw-Hill Education; 2011.

9. Santana R, Rosemary A. Need, demand, supply in health care: Working definitions, and their implications for defining access. [cited 2022 Oct 5]. Available from: https://doi.org/10.1017/S1744133121000293

10. Leal JR, Conly J, Henderson EA, Manns BJ. How externalities impact an evaluation of strategies to prevent antimicrobial resistance in health care organizations. Antimicrob Resist Infect Control [Internet]. 2017 Jun 2 [cited 2022 Oct 5];6(1):1–11. Available from: https://link.springer.com/articles/10.1186/s13756-017-0211-2

11. Drummond M, Sculpher MJ, Claxton K, Stoddart GL, Torrance GW, Askews & Holts Library Services. Methods for the economic evaluation of health care programmes [Internet]. [cited 2020 Sep 7]. 445 p. Available from: https://books.google.co.in/books?hl=en&lr=&id=yzZSCwAAQBAJ&oi=fnd&pg=PP1&dq=drummond+economic+evaluation&ots=_aVjlH9uEP&sig=2C16aHFHHM_6Jb9g5nZXq674_gs&redir_esc=y#v=onepage&q=drummond economic evaluation&f=false

12. Brown H. The economics of public health: Evaluating public health interventions. Econ Public Heal Eval Public Heal Interv. 2018 Apr 12;1–107.

13. Drummond M, Stoddart G, Labelle R, Cushman R. Health economics: An introduction for clinicans. Ann Intern Med. 1987;107(1):88–92.

14. Dolan P. Modeling valuations for EuroQol Health States. Med Care [Internet]. 1997 Jan 10;35(11):1095–108. Available from: www.jstor.org/stable/3767472

15. Gothwal VK, Bagga DK. Utility values in the visually impaired: Comparing time-trade off and visqol. Optom Vis Sci [Internet]. 2013 Aug [cited 2022 Sep 30];90(8):843–54. Available from: https://journals.lww.com/optvissci/Fulltext/2013/08000/Utility_Values_in_the_Visually_Impaired__Comparing.16.aspx

16. Larson BA. Calculating disability-adjusted-life-years lost (DALYs) in discrete-time. Cost Eff Resour Alloc. 2013;11(1):18.

17. Byford S, Torgerson DJ, Raftery J. Economic note: Cost of illness studies. BMJ [Internet]. 2000 May 13 [cited 2020 May 31];320(7245):1335. Available from: www.ncbi.nlm.nih.gov/pubmed/10807635

18. Jo C. Cost-of-illness studies: Concepts, scopes, and methods. Clin Mol Hepatol [Internet]. 2014 Dec 1 [cited 2022 Sep 27];20(4):327. Available from: /pmc/articles/PMC4278062/

19. Tarricone R. Cost-of-illness analysis. What room in health economics? Health Policy (New York). 2006 Jun;77(1):51–63.

20. Green D, Ducorroy G, McElnea E, Naughton A, Skelly A, O'Neill C, et al. The cost of blindness in the Republic of Ireland 2010–2020. J Ophthalmol [Internet]. 2016 [cited 2020 Apr 6];2016:1–8. Available from: www.hindawi. com/journals/joph/2016/4691276/

21. Rein DB, Wittenborn JS, Zhang P, Sublett F, Lamuda PA, Lundeen EA, et al. The economic burden of vision loss and blindness in the United States. Ophthalmology. 2022 Apr 1;129(4):369–78.

22. Köberlein J, Beifus K, Schaffert C, Finger RP. The economic burden of visual impairment and blindness: A systematic review. BMJ Open [Internet]. 2013 Nov 7 [cited 2020 Apr 2];3(11):e003471. Available from: www.ncbi.nlm.nih. gov/pubmed/24202057

23. Burton MJ, Ramke J, Marques AP, Bourne RRA, Congdon N, Jones I, et al. The Lancet Global Health Commission on Global Eye Health: Vision beyond 2020. Lancet Glob Heal [Internet]. 2021 Apr 1 [cited 2022 Sep 27];9(4):e489–551. Available from: www.thelancet.com/article/ S2214109X20304885/fulltext

24. Mannava S, Borah R, Shamanna B. Current estimates of the economic burden of blindness and visual impairment in India: A cost of illness study. Indian J Ophthalmol [Internet]. 2022 [cited 2022 Jun 13];70(6):2141. Available from: https://journals.lww.com/ijo/Fulltext/2022/06000/Current_ estimates_of_the_economic_burden_of.53.aspx

25. Wong B, Singh K, Khanna RK, Ravilla T, Sabherwal S, Sil A, et al. The Economic and Social Cost of Visual Impairment and Blindness in India [Internet]. 2021 [cited 2022 Sep 10]. Available from: www.seva.org/site/ DocServer/Seva_Cost_of_Visual_Impairment_in_India.pdf

26. Köberlein J, Beifus K, Schaffert C, Finger RP. The economic burden of visual impairment and blindness: A systematic review. BMJ Open. 2013;3(11).

27. Byford S, Torgerson DJ, Raftery J. Cost of illness studies. BMJ [Internet]. 2000 May 13 [cited 2022 Sep 27];320(7245):1335. Available from: www.bmj. com/content/320/7245/1335.1

28. Bourne RRA, Steinmetz JD, Flaxman S, Briant PS, Taylor HR, Resnikoff S, et al. Trends in prevalence of blindness and distance and near vision impairment over 30 years: An analysis for the Global Burden of Disease Study. Lancet Glob Heal [Internet]. 2021 Feb 1 [cited 2022 Sep 26];9(2):e130–43. Available from: www.thelancet.com/article/ S2214109X20304253/fulltext

29. WHO | What is VISION 2020? [cited 2015 Aug 24]. Available from: www. who.int/blindness/partnerships/vision2020/en/

30. Bertram MY, Edejer TTT. Introduction to the special issue on "The World Health Organization choosing interventions that are cost-effective (WHO-CHOICE) update." Int J Heal Policy Manag [Internet]. 2021 Nov 1 [cited 2022 Sep 30];10 (Special Issue on WHO-CHOICE Update):670–2. Available from: www.ijhpm.com/article_4139.html

31. Husereau D, Drummond M, Augustovski F, de Bekker-Grob E, Briggs AH, Carswell C, et al. Consolidated Health Economic Evaluation Reporting Standards 2022 (CHEERS 2022) statement: Updated reporting guidance for health economic evaluations. Heal Policy OPEN. 2022 Dec 1;3.

11

Low Vision and Rehabilitation

SURAJ SINGH SENJAM, SOUVIK MANNA,
PRAVEEN VASHIST

LEARNING OBJECTIVES

At the end of this chapter, the reader will be able to:

1. Learn the basics of defining *low vision* and *blindness*.
2. Enhance skills in caring for the people who require vision rehabilitation.
3. Learn how to establish low-vision and rehabilitation clinics in areas where they are needed.

11.1 DEFINITION

11.1.1 Definitions of Vision Loss

Any person having presenting visual acuity in better eye ≤6/18–3/60 is defined as low vision as per WHO definition. Such persons are the beneficiaries of low-vision rehabilitation services. Low-vision rehabilitation (LVR) is the process of restoring functional ability and improving quality of life and independence of a patient with low vision. It requires a thorough clinical and functional assessment of the disease, of patients' requirements and daily needs. Thereafter, the rehabilitation is tailored to correspond to the type of the visual disability and the individual's expectations.

11.1.2 Prevention of Low Vision

There may be one or more causes of low vision. These are usually the result of disorders or injuries affecting the eye or a disorder such as diabetes that affects the entire body. Some of the most common causes of low vision include age-related macular degeneration, diabetes, and glaucoma. Low vision may also result from

DOI: 10.1201/9781003291626-11

Table 11.1 Definitions of Vision Loss

Categories	Presenting Visual Acuity in Better Eye
Normal vision	6/6–6/12
Low vision (WHO definition)	6/18–3/60
Welfare definition of legal blindness	<6/60
EVI (early visual impairment/mild VI)	<6/12–6/18
MVI (moderate visual impairment)	<6/18–6/60
SVI (severe visual impairment)	<6/60–3/60
WHO definition of blindness	<3/60

cancer of the eye, albinism, brain injury, or inherited disorders of the eye, including retinitis pigmentosa.

Some sight disorders, like diabetic retinopathy, can be treated to restore or maintain vision. When this is not possible, low vision is permanent. However, many people with low vision find visual aids helpful. Popular low-vision aids include telescopic glasses, lenses that filter light, magnifying glasses, hand magnifiers, closed-circuit television, and reading prisms.

In some patients, the restored vision allows for them to independently navigate through doorways and sidewalks, sort light- and dark-coloured laundry, or even read large letters. Non-optical aids designed for people with low vision are also very helpful. Some popular non-optical devices include text-reading software, check guides, high-contrast clocks and watches, talking watches and clocks, large-print publications, clocks, phones- and watches with enlarged numbers. Visual aids improve both sight and the quality of life for many people.

Low vision may be preventable for patients with diabetes, and some patients with macular degeneration and glaucoma may be treated to prevent the further vision loss.

11.1.3 CBR (Community-Based Rehabilitation) Matrix and ICF Framework

The International Classification of Impairments, Disabilities, and Handicaps (ICIDH-I), the World Health Organization, in the 1980s, defines *disability* as any restriction or lack of ability resulting from an impairment in performing any activity within the range considered normal for a human being. This definition explains the very nature of the medical model of disability, in which *disability* is considered as purely a medical problem or body impairment on account of disease. However, in 2001, the ICIDH-II, now named as ICF (the International Classification of Functioning, Disability, and Health), recommends that disability should no longer be viewed as merely the result of anatomical impairment or diseases, rather viewed as the umbrella term with impairments, activity limitations, and participation restrictions, and as a consequence of negative interaction of these components within the individual's socio-environment context.

Caring for a person with low vision is challenging for most caregivers. *Special needs* is an umbrella term that refers to an array of diagnoses and disabilities. It is used to identify mental, physical, and psychological disabilities that affect a person's function and behaviour (1). A study on expectations of patients prior to attending the LV clinic reported new spectacles (47%), magnifiers or LV devices (27%), advice/explanation of medical condition (13%), CCTV/electronic magnification system (7%), large print (7%), help using computer (7%), "morale boost" (7%), and cataract surgery (7%) as the most common reasons for visit (2). The effectiveness of low-vision rehabilitation have been demonstrated in both children and adults (3, 4).

The ability to use vision is very important for independent functioning and performing most behaviour within each developmental area. Holding objects, looking at and smiling at the caregiver, manipulating toys, searching for the hidden toys and objects, playing with the peers, etc. are affected by visual impairment.

When the child is born, the visual capacity of the child is very limited. The visual sense is the least-developed sense at birth, although this sense organ is the first to be formed in foetal life.

Significance of vision in different areas of development:

1. *Motor development.* Surprisingly, children with visual problems tend to achieve some of the milestones of motor development at about the same time and in the same sequence as the other infants. However, they show considerable delay in achieving self-initiated mobility and in reaching for objects.
2. *Cognitive development.* Spatial relationship, spatial orientation, imitation of verbal and gesture language, discrimination of size, shape, colour, and identification of objects are the concepts that develop faster with the help of vision.
3. *Social development.* Visually impaired infants and toddlers have very immature social behaviours and inappropriate play and interaction patterns and hence are less likely to make friends easily. The lack of effective interpersonal skills has a lifelong impact on leisure time activities and success in jobs.
4. *Play development.* Visually impaired children are delayed in exploring the environment and objects. They are less likely to engage in elaborate play routines. Other characteristics of play in visually challenged infants are failure to use their hands to reach and explore objects and later development of imitation of actions and play routines.
5. *Speech and language development.* Usually, language acquisition in children with visual impairment is not affected, but markable delay in certain aspects is noted.

Low-vision dispensing is a new, emerging subspecialty drawing from the traditional fields of ophthalmology, optometry, occupational therapy, and sociology, with an ever-increasing impact on our customary concepts of research, education, and services for the visually impaired and blind patient. It helps practitioners ensure that practitioners put patients' interests first and work in partnership with them so they receive the best possible care.

The government of India has launched the ADIP scheme for assistance to low-vision children in obtaining various assistive devices (5). The dispensing of optical, non-optical electronic devices to patients who are registered as sight-impaired or severely sight-impaired must be carried out by or under the supervision of the practitioner. Advice on visual efficiency and comfort should include reading posture, reading stand, copy holders, clipboards, and higher reading additions. Practitioners should consider binocularity and accommodation when dispensing a patient with any device. Before dispensing any device, the practitioner should assess patients carrying out relevant practical tasks with the device to identify any limitations. The overall purpose of LVR is to maximize access to printed material, improve ability to accomplish ADL and perform tasks of interest, improve safety, optimize social participation, improve psychological status and adjustment to vision loss, and enhance awareness of options for psychological support with overall improvement in quality of life (6). The importance of going beyond regular VA testing for children with low vision in clinical practice is highly recommended. With patience, suitably adapted methods, a familiar environment, and skill, visual assessment is feasible in the majority of children with special needs (7).

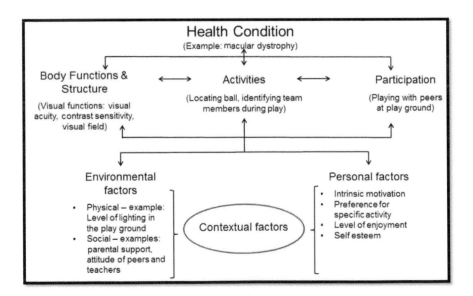

Figure 11.1 The International Classification of Functioning, Disability, and Health framework.

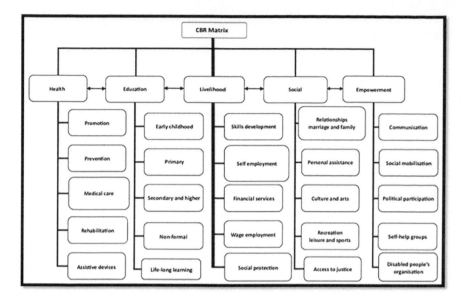

Figure 11.2 The Community-Based Rehabilitation matrix.

11.2 ORIENTATION AND MOBILITY

11.2.1 Self- and Independent Movements

The focus of self- and independent movement is usually to perform all kinds of indoor activities, for example, to do daily and routine activities, like going to toilets, bathroom, bed; using stairs; etc. The training is usually provided as one-to-one. Self- and independent mobility is the first step in learning for all people with visual loss. Motivation, encouragement, building confidence to the clients are key initial steps. Regular practice is important for efficient and smooth movement. Correct positioning of arm, forearm, and figure is essential in self- and independent mobility.

11.2.2 Human or Sighted

Human guide is a technique where a person with visual impairment takes help from someone with sight as a guide in movement form one place to another. The guide gives the verbal cues or instructions while navigating, and the client follows the cues accordingly.

11.2.3 Mobility Using Walking Long Cane

People with visual loss need other sense of the body to be able to travel safely, effectively, and independently at outside environment. Mobility cane is the most important mobility tool which helps in outdoor movement in both familiar and unfamiliar settings. The best way to provide orientation and mobility training is one-to-one manner or into a small group of clients. Before the start of mobility training, iden-tification of important landmarks and location of person in relation to his or her environment is a fundamental aspect for travelling using long walking cane.

11.2.4 Activities of Daily Living

Activities of daily living (ADLs) are basic tasks that must be accomplished every day for an individual to thrive. Generally, ADLs can be broken down into the fol-lowing categories:

11.2.4.1 PERSONAL HYGIENE

Bathing, grooming, oral, nail, and hair care.

11.2.4.2 CONTINENCE MANAGEMENT

A person's mental and physical ability to properly use the bathroom.

11.2.4.3 DRESSING

A person's ability to select and wear the proper clothes for different occasions.

11.2.4.4 FEEDING

Whether a person can feed themselves or needs assistance.

11.2.4.5 AMBULATING

The extent of a person's ability to change from one position to another and to walk independently.

11.2.5 Smartphones for Low-Vision Rehabilitation

A *smartphone* is a specialized phone with multipurpose functions. A smartphone that uses Android or iOS operating system will give the user access to apps that have been specially designed for visually impaired users (text-magnification apps or text-to-speech apps). People with visual disability get more out of such a smartphone.

Application (app). A computer programme with a specific purpose and func-tion, for example, WhatsApp and Instagram, designed to run on smartphones and tablets. For a person with poor or no eyesight, using a mobile phone can be a chal-lenge. And yet a mobile phone, particularly a smartphone, is now omnipresent and has become an essential part of life for everyone in doing everyday activities.

Frequently Used Applications

1. Be My Eyes
2. VISOR
3. EYE D Pro

4. SUPERSENSE
5. TapTapSee
6. MANI
7. Google Assistant
8. Talk Back
9. Select to Speak
10. Magnify Screen
11. Binoculars

11.3 COMMUNITY-BASED REHABILITATION AND PRIMARY EYE CARE

Primary eye care (PEC) is a broad concept, encompassing the prevention of potentially blinding eye diseases through primary health centres (PHC). *Primary eye care* is defined as "a 'frontline' activity, providing eye care and identifying disease before it becomes a serious medical issue." It is aimed at eye health promotion and early identification with timely referral of people with ocular morbidity. Primary-level health worker or volunteers can help in the prevention and control of blindness by eye health promotion in the community, creating awareness about the blinding conditions, identification of common eye conditions, and referral to higher-level eye care centres. Primary eye care is aimed at eye care promotion through behaviour change in the community, community awareness, and participation needs to be strengthened at the grassroots level in order to identify and treat individuals with ocular morbidity within the community. PEC can be successful in a programme setting when it is integrated in the existing health systems and establishes linkages with other associated sectors, such as education, water resources, and social welfare, to enable eye health promotion.

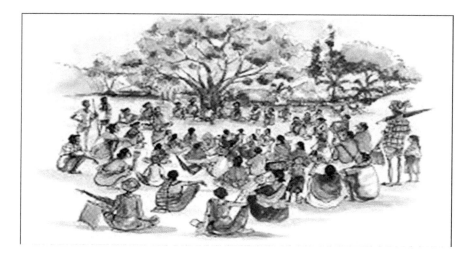

Figure 11.3 A pictogram depicting a village self-help group for empowering vulnerable persons.

More than 80% of blindness and 90% of visual impairment are either preventable or curable. One of the reasons for such high level of avoidable blindness in the country is poorly accessible eye care services to a large proportion of people. Majority of eye care services are concentrated in urban areas. There is a high level of poverty and illiteracy in the rural population that is responsible for poor awareness about the prevention and treatment of eye diseases, which in turn is responsible for under-utilization of available eye care services. It is essential that primary eye care services be available at the doorstep to the people in rural areas, in order to reduce the burden of blindness.

One major hindrance to achieving universal PEC is that in developing countries, especially from South-East Asian region, full-time eye care workforce is extremely insufficient. In all countries, the primary care workers formally employed by the public health system have the responsibilities to conduct house visits and conduct primary eye care, although the eye care component is often neglected in favour of delivering reproductive health and communicable disease control services. There is also a disproportionate distribution of these workforces between rural and urban area.

One way to overcome this challenge is to solicit a proactive role of volunteers in primary eye care. In many South Asian countries, community members are volunteering in projects through NGOs (non-governmental organizations), such as the Shastho Shebikas introduced by the NGO BRAC (Bangladesh Rehabilitation Assistance Committee). In Nepal, there are female community health volunteers, who are working under the government ambit. In India, ASHA (accredited social health activist) has brought an exemplary change in primary health care accessibility by being a successful link worker between the community and the health centres. In addition, multiple NGOs have successfully built models for involving eye care volunteers. In Sri Lanka, there are no volunteers formally engaged by the health system. Often, non-formal volunteerism also takes place by way of using school teachers and community members in eye care activities. Before volunteers can actually deliver primary eye care, they must receive a comprehensive sensitization and training so that they get equipped with the requisite knowledge and skills to provide primary eye care services at the grassroots level.

An important component of PEC is vision rehabilitation for persons with visual disability. The components that are of paramount importance for vision rehabilitation are summarized in the CBR matrix, that is, health, education, livelihood, social rehabilitation, and empowerment. Under the health component is the entire gamut of services including promotive, preventive, curative, rehabilitative, and palliative (assistive technology). Improving access to assistive technologies is also included under the health component of the CBR matrix. Under the education component, the rehabilitation worker needs to address the needs of patients starting from early childhood, primary, secondary, and higher education. Those who are unable to accommodate themselves in mainstream schooling need to be provided avenues for non-formal education. Finally, it is also important to imbibe a culture of lifelong learning in all persons with disability, as learning is seldom complete, even after formal education. Under the livelihood component, avenues like skills development, self-employment, wage employment, and various financial services are included. Persons with disability must be abreast with the various financial and social protection schemes by the government to lead an independent and dignified life. Under social rehabilitation, there are avenues like marriage, relationship, family life, personal assistance, learning about arts and culture, recreation, leisure, sports, and access to judicial system. The entire gamut of social services must be available to persons with disabilities without any discrimination. The most important component is empowerment, which includes communication, social mobilization, political participation, and the ability to participate in SHG (self-help groups) and DPOs (disabled persons organizations).

REFERENCES

1. Helen Chan. Understanding Children with Special Needs. Caremark [Internet]. 2019 [cited 2020 Oct 22]. Available from: www.caremark.ie/understanding-children-with-special-needs/
2. Crossland MD, Gould ES, Helman CG, Feely MP, Rubin GS. Expectations and perceived benefits of a hospital-based low vision clinic: Results of an exploratory, qualitative research study. Vis Impair Res. 2007;9(2–3):59–66.
3. Gothwal VK, Sumalini R, Bharani S. Assessing the effectiveness of low Vision Rehabilitation in children: An observational study. Investig Ophthalmol Vis Sci. 2015;56(5):3355–60.
4. Stelmack JA, Tang XC, Wei Y, Massof RW. The effectiveness of low-vision rehabilitation in 2 cohorts derived from the veterans affairs Low-Vision Intervention Trial. Arch Ophthalmol (Chicago, Ill 1960). 2012 Sep;130(9):1162–8.
5. ADIP Scheme—Vikaspedia [Internet]. [cited 2020 Mar 12]. Available from: https://vikaspedia.in/social-welfare/differently-abled-welfare/schemes-programmes/adip-scheme
6. Fontenot JL, Bona MD, Kaleem MA, McLaughlin WM, Morse AR, Schwartz TL, et al. Vision rehabilitation preferred practice pattern®. Ophthalmology. 2018;125(1):P228–78.
7. Das M, Spowart K, Crossley S, Dutton GN. Evidence that children with special needs all require visual assessment. Arch Dis Child. 2010;95(11):888–92.

12

Management of Low Vision

SUMIT GROVER, MONICA CHAUDHARY,
SURAJ SINGH SENJAM

12.1 UNDERSTANDING LOW VISION

A person with low vision is the one who has impairment of visual functions even after treatment or standard refractive correction and has visual acuity of less than 6/18 or a visual field less than 10 degrees from the point of fixation but is the one who uses or is potentially able to use vision for planning and execution of task.

Low vision is based on functional definition and functional disability factors, such that loss of vision interferes with daily activities, occupation, recreation, and social interaction. In simpler words, it is vision loss which is not correctable by glasses, contact lenses, medicine, and surgery and impacts the functional abilities of a patient. Low-vision rehabilitation is an integral part of low-vision eye exam, as the low-vision devices prescribed for rehabilitation maximizes visual functionality. Management of low vision is a team approach; it includes ophthalmologists, optometrists, occupational therapists, rehabilitative counsellors, psychological service providers, and special educators.

The management of low vision comprises four phases:

1. Identifying the needs and functional difficulties
2. Evaluation of the patient
3. Recommending low-vision devices
4. Rehabilitation

To summarize, *low vision* is partial sight which makes an individual have some disabilities, and the management is simply to make them functional and independent.

12.2 CAUSES OF LOW VISION

Ocular pathologies which lead to irreversible, non-treatable damage to the eye result in low vision. The common disorders in children for low vision are albinism,

138

DOI: 10.1201/9781003291626-12

optic neuropathy, trauma, congenital malformations, corneal opacity, and amblyopia. In young adults, the loss of vision is late onset of congenital disorders or trauma. In old age, the most common cause is age-related macular degeneration, glaucoma, myopic degeneration, or diabetic retinopathy.

12.3 EXAMINING THE LOW-VISION PATIENT

12.3.1 Goals of Low-Vision Management

Increase functionality; make the most of the remaining vision.
Provide link to community resources and support services.
Health education and awareness.
Complete ocular and systemic clinical assessment.

12.3.2 Assessment of Needs

Assessment should be focused on the impact of disease on the functionality in terms of vision disability for distance, near, vocational, occupational, or specific demands of the patients.

- Extent of vision: near and distance visual acuity.
- Size of the visual field.
- Effect of light and glare.
- Extent of recognition and naming of colour.
- Extent to which contrast affects their activities.
- Extent of use of vision for different activities and purpose in the environment.
- Extent to which a person sees and recognizes an object depends, among others, on familiarity of the object, light, size, distance, contrast, colour, detail or simplicity of the object.
- Age, socioeconomic conditions, literacy status, and level of motivation.

The examination of the low-vision patient begins in the waiting area, where the eye care practitioner observes and understands the mobility and the severity of the visual impairment by observation as the patient enters the clinic.

12.3.3 History Taking

The history taking begins with reviewing the medical records and a quick understanding of the treatment process the patient has gone through. The low-vision exam begins only after the best possible medical surgical or optical treatment has been accomplished so far; hence, time should not be wasted on re-examinations. The evaluation in low-vision clinic is beyond, by making the patient functional and augmenting the residual vision.

There are a series of questions which allow rapid screening to the practitioner to understand the needs so that proper devices can be recommended, followed by rehabilitation services.

Examples of a few of the questions to understand disability for distance are: Do you have problems walking around? Do you take assistance when you go outdoors? How is your mobility indoors and in your familiar surroundings? How comfortable are you in identifying faces, recognizing people, and handling your daily routines independently? How do you manage your free time watching television? Are you comfortable sitting close and watching? Can you sign your name? Etc.

The questions are related to the age, occupation, and requirement of the patient. For example, for a school-going student, the questions would refer to blackboard copying, reading, writing. One needs to ask about the size of the print that they usually refer to. For an old person sitting at home, the questions will be addressed more to independence and recreation. For an employee working on computers, the questions will refer to all related to computer or office work.

Assessment of need for enhanced illumination or preference towards low light is asked so that it can be integrated into the management plan. Several disorders lead to glare problem and reduced vision quality. For various diseases, patients have issues with contrast and hence reduced functioning in low illumination. Understanding preferences during history taking helps in the right suggestion of devices to boost quality of vision.

Assessment of mental health should be integrated in a low-vision exam as far as possible. Most of visually impaired patients are either anxious or depressed. Mental health and psychological counselling are as valuable for the reason that failures are seen without managing psychological well-being. If the patient doesn't have acceptance of the disorder or disability prior to the dispensing of low-vision devices, the patient will not acknowledge your recommendations. Visual impairment not only impacts an individual but also has influences on the family, specially the caregiver, whose life has been moulded to serve the patient. One needs to understand this socioeconomic impact and suggest the right direction by this through rehabilitation services.

12.3.4 Vision Assessment for Distance and Near

Estimating visual acuity, the best corrected visual acuity is important for magnification calculation of optical devices. The assessment is not only on quantity of vision but also on quality of vision, which relates to contrast sensitivity and glare acuity.

The acuity recording is different than the regular Snellen's charts. While measuring acuity counting, finger documentation is not the right way of recording the visual acuity in these patients. The clinic should have logMAR charts for distances and near (Figure 12.1). These charts are made for use for 4 m. However, if visual acuity is lesser, the chart is brought closer to half the distance, that is 2 m, or still

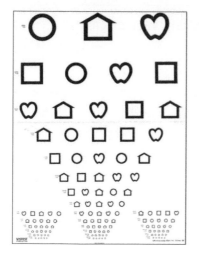 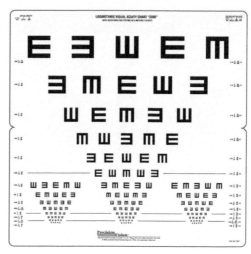

Figure 12.1 LogMAR charts used in low-vision assessment.

closer to 1 m in severe impairments. The visual equity can be easily converted for 2 m or 1 m distance.

Recording near visual acuity is also done with special low-vision charts. The M unit notation and 1 M later subtends 5 min of arc at 1 m. The recording example is 1 M or 2 M @ 40 cm. These M unit acuity charts assist in calculating the magnification. Suppose a patient reads 2 M at 40 cm; to read 1 M size, they would need 2× magnification. These charts are simple calculators of the magnification and help make the preparation for trial of devices simple.

12.3.5 Refraction

The method of refraction is both objective and subjective. The retinoscopy findings are superior and a better starting point than autorefractor readings. Subjective testing is done with appropriate distance chart 1 m, 2 m, or 4 m, and the bracketing technique is used. If the glow is not clear radical retinoscopy, that means going closer than even 50 cm is recommended to have some rough understanding of the refractive error. Patients with 6/60 visual acuity will not appreciate small changes of 0.25 or 0.5 dioptre; therefore, larger step changes should be done in subjective refinement. Cross cylinders also of one dioptre value are used. Patient usually has a habitual glass and refining power over these glasses, followed by instinctively making the patient look around in the room, comparing the quality of vision with current glasses and the new prescription. One should assess the functional vision by moving beyond the visual acuity charts and understanding the vision quantity by looking at objects around.

Contrast sensitivity can be measured by any standard chart, like the Pelli–Robson (Figure 12.2). Questions to understand the reduced contrast in daily routine may be added. Enhancing illumination for daily activities is added as

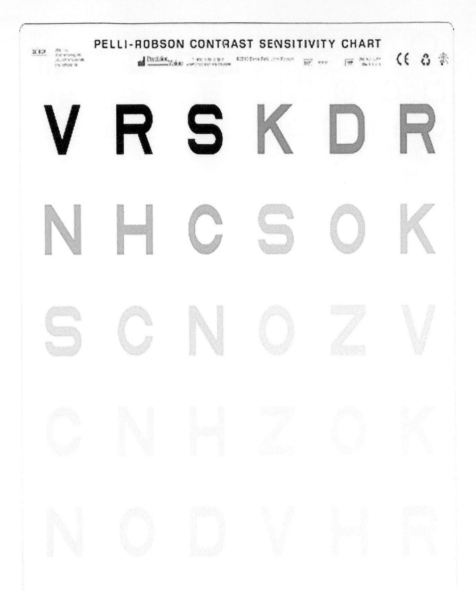

Figure 12.2 Pelli–Robson contrast sensitivity chart.

management to all patients who document poor contrast. Discussion about preferences on task and its lighting is done during assessment.

Visual field assessment. A low-vision patient should be categorized into various types of field defects. The management plan differs, depending upon the field loss found. Broadly, it is classified as central field loss or peripheral field loss. Besides this, a patient may have scotomas, hemianopia, or overall blurred vision. Goldman perimetry is still considered to be best; however, it is not readily available in all clinics. The recommendation is to have a quick screening of visual fields by confrontation testing and assessing the central visual field with Amsler's charts. Automated perimeters may not be the best choice for these patients; however, kinetic perimetry can give a fair extent of field loss in Humphrey or Octopus perimeters. A good understanding about the visual field of the patient, his preferences and his gaze position, is important to prescribe devices.

12.4 MANAGEMENT OF LOW VISION WITH DEVICES

A low-vision aid refers to an optical device which improves or enhances residual vision by magnifying the image of the object. The calculation of magnification forms the basis of any low-vision optical/non-optical device.

1. *Relative distance magnification.* Simply by taking the object closer to the eye, it will appear bigger.
2. *Angular magnification.* Use of hand magnifiers, stand magnifiers, or telescopes falls under this category.
3. *Relative size magnification.* Making the object larger, like making the textbook print size larger, is an example of this magnification.

It is categorized into two broader classifications:

1. Optical devices
2. Non-optical devices

Recent advances of electronic devices can be classified into an additional third group.

12.4.1 Optical Devices

Broadly, optical devices are of four types:

1. Spectacle magnifiers
2. Hand magnifiers
3. Stand magnifiers
4. Telescopes

Further, they can be divided into:

1. Distance, which includes telescopes (Figure 12.3)
2. Near, which includes spectacle magnifiers, handheld magnifiers, and stand magnifiers as optical devices (Figure 12.4)

Magnifying spectacles. These are the most commonly prescribed low-vision devices and can be given in a basic set-up of refraction room also. They are

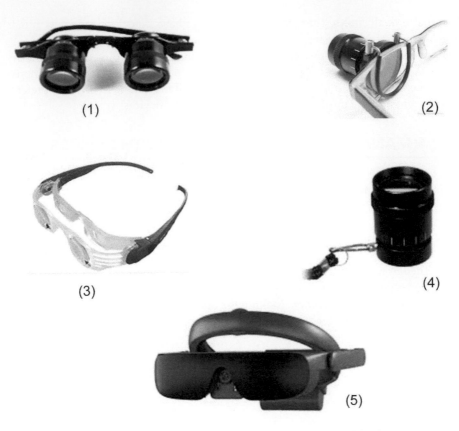

Figure 12.3 Optical aids for distance correction: (1) a handheld telescope, (2) spectacle-mounted telescope, (3) TV glasses, (4) clip-on telescope, (5) iris vision.

prescribed for near and work on the simple principle of magnification by a convex lens. When the object is placed at the focal length of this convex lens, it creates an erect magnified image. For a high-plus lens mounted in a standard full frame or half frame, the powers range from anything beyond 4 dioptres. These are useful as the hands are free; the disadvantage is that one must hold it at the focal point, which is usually very close to the eye. The reading distance of a 10-dioptre magnifier would be 10 cm, and of +5 would be 20 cm. The reading at close distance is the major disadvantage; however, slant reading tables and others can be added along to improve posture; the advantages include convenience and both hands being free.

Handheld magnifiers. These magnifying devices produce a virtual image, and the reading material is held at the focal length of the magnifying lens. The image is produced at infinity and hence magnifies. These devices are illuminated or non-illuminated, available in various powers starting from 2× magnification. Usual prescriptions range below 8× magnification, because the size of the optical lens

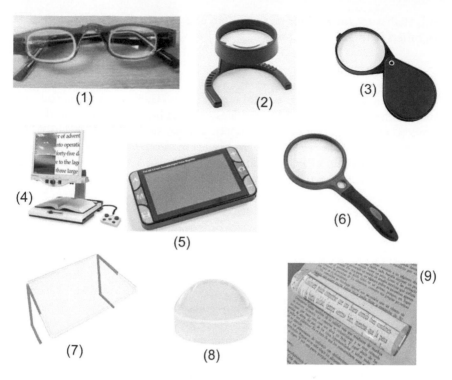

Figure 12.4 Optical aids for near correction: (1) spectacle magnifier, (2) stand magnifier, (3) pocket magnifier, (4) desktop magnifier, (5) video magnifier, (6) handheld magnifier, (7) Fresnel Sheet, (8) dome magnifier, (9) bar magnifier.

reduces as magnification is increased. The benefits of these are, it is used for reading or any near activity for a short while. It can be combined with other spectacle magnifiers, and the eye can have a normal reading distance. These are easily available and are less-expensive. Patients can use eccentric viewing, specially in field defects. Adding illumination or having self-illuminated magnifiers improves the contrast and is the most convenient portable device. It is difficult to be used in old patients with poor manual dexterity, and the patient must hold the object at the right focal distance throughout the reading, hence needs steady focus and keeps the hand occupied.

Stand magnifier. Similar to hand magnifiers, stand magnifiers produce an enlarged virtual image in front of the eye, and hence, the patient uses his near prescription and keeps the material at the focal length of the lens for reading. The device is recommended in patients with field effects and poor manual dexterity. It is helpful in schoolchildren, specially with central field loss, as they can use their eccentric viewing and peep through the magnifier to get added advantage of magnification. The major disadvantage of these devices is reduced field of vision and poor posture of reading. Stand magnifiers are recommended to be used with a reading stand. They require a flat surface to read. Higher magnifications can be given, and illumination is added in these magnifiers to increase the contrast.

12.4.2 Telescopes

Telescopes in low vision are usually of two types: Galilean or Keplerian. The Galilean telescope has a plus objective lens in a minus eyepiece. Most of the prescriptions are Galilean telescope prescriptions because they produce an upright, erect image and are simpler designs and smaller in size.

The telescopes can be monocular or binocular. The advantages are that the patient can view far-off things easily by holding it in hand or by attaching it in the spectacles. Telescope prescriptions are usually given in school-going children who intend to see blackboards. Advancement in designs has happened, and sleeker models are now available for adults which are cosmetically appealing. Also, higher magnifications reduce the field of vision, and hence, telescopes are usually within the range of 6× magnification.

A Keplerian telescope has a larger field of vision and can be given in higher magnification but has an inverted image, for which a prism is added into the optics. These are a little more complicated designs and sometimes are difficult to handle.

CCTV or electronic systems. There are many low-vision devices now which incorporate electronic systems for magnifying. These devices have a reasonable field of view and can be given up to 40× magnification. The reading distance is also comfortable compared to other optical devices, and it has several other features which enhance the quality of vision. These devices are expensive for many of our patients.

To summarize, there are several shapes and types of these broadly classified magnifiers—dome magnifier, bar magnifier, clip-on monocular telescopes, bioptic telescopes, LED stand magnifiers, LED hand magnifiers, etc.—made available by various manufacturers in various powers and designs. The choice of shape and type of these magnifiers is totally based on patients' requirements and outcomes. Several contrast-enhancing and glare-cutting filters also add on enhancement of the visual acuity.

The selection of the device depends upon the patient's need, and both quality and quantity of vision costs are sometimes a matter of concern along with the motivation. There are several electronic devices, like smartphones and computer software, which make objects larger and can even enhance contrast. Technologies have enhanced over the last decades, and there are several assistive technologies, like text-to-speech readers, and smartphone apps that function like low-vision devices.

12.4.3 Non-Optical Devices

Non-optical devices do not rely on optical lenses for enhancing magnification but rather use relative size illumination increasing contrast or other sensory inputs for enhancing the effects. They are mostly integrated with optical devices to enhance functionality (Figure 12.5).

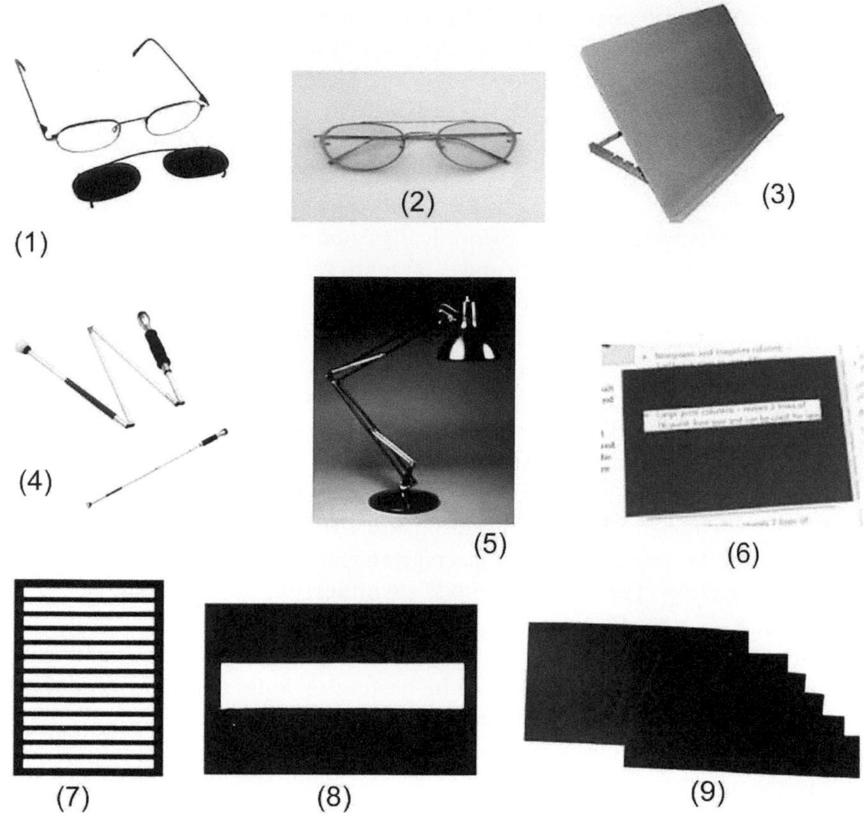

Figure 12.5 Non-optical devices used in low vision: (1) clip-on glasses, (2) amber filter glasses, (3) reading stand, (4) canes, (5) reading Lamp, (6) typo-scope, (7) letter writing guide, (8) signature guide, (9) Notex.

Categorizing a few examples of non-optical device prescriptions are as follows:

1. Using large-size objects or large print. Font size 14 to 24 books are available globally. National curriculum textbooks are also available for visually impaired in large print size. If not available, the books can be scanned, photocopied, and printed out in a larger size. The disadvantage is bulkiness of these books. Other examples of such devices are recommending large-size telephone or a watch with bigger-size print. The advantage is, one does not need an additional optical device to magnify and identify the object.

2. Enhancing illumination by using table lamps, reading lamps. Patients with cataract glaucoma and RP are broadly bothered by poor contrast. Enhancing illumination by using fluorescent light, halogen light, or neo-dymium bulb helps these patients.

3. Albinism, aniridia, rod cone dystrophy, and RP patients are sensitive to outdoor lighting, and it's a source of glare for them. Using peak caps and

glasses with side shield reduce both glare and enhance contrast. There are special filters to enhance. Special filters are developed by various standard companies which reduce photophobia and glare. These are special transmittance, flame filters, UV protective too. A polarized filter reduces glare from reflecting surfaces. Anti-reflection coatings are not much of an advantage; however, the mirror coatings can reduce transmittance by absorption and reflection.

4. Pinhole spectacles are more theoretically important or can be attempted in patients with corneal opacity and cataract to reduce blur.

5. Adjustment of appropriate colour in contrast in the working environment. Making the colour of walls and furniture a strong contrast to that of doors and windows, handles, edges of staircases, etc. helps a patient enhance functionality. The contrast in the kitchen can be enhanced by making combinations of light and dark objects, for example, pouring milk in a dark cup and pouring tea in a light cup.

6. Slant reading tables. These are posture enhancers that bring comfort to patients who bend close to do reading and writing. They are a must prescription for patients who have been given stand magnifiers.

7. Reading lamp. The reading lamp is a wonderful non-optical device which enhances contrast, and almost every patient who needs brighter illumination and has poor contrast shows significant advantage of using reading lamps. The lamp should be preferably long, and light should not fall on the eye. The paper should not be glossy to reflect and cause glare issues; white or yellow light preference can be discussed and prescribed to the patient.

8. Signature guide. Signing by oneself is sometimes an issue with severe visual impairment. The signature guide has a small cut-out in a black heart paper, and it facilitates signatures by guiding him through the blurred vision the patient has.

9. Reading guide or typoscope. Patients are unable to orient their reading and comprehend from one line to another. Using a typoscope guides them to read through a straight line and even eliminates contrast and glare.

10. Writing guides are cut-outs of these lines in a black cardboard, like a folder. They are recommended to elderly or children for writing comfort.

11. Other daily activity assistive technologies, such as using large prints, range monitoring, blood sugar monitoring, blood pressure with readout, thermometers, talking thermometers, etc., are freely available online, and patients can buy these products depending on their needs.

12. Mobility and orientation. Mobility drops significantly in severely visually impaired patients. Talking books, talking calculators, watches, computers, and telephones are part of non-optical devices.

13. Especially for ones with peripheral field loss, gains or special mobility devices are trained by the rehabilitation centre's guide by using tactile, hearing, touch, and other substitutions. There are several devices available in the market.

14. Guide dogs. It is an organization which trains these dogs to assist visually impaired persons.

12.5 ORIENTATION AND MOBILITY TRAINING

Objectives of orientation and mobility training:

- *Safety*. To move around safe and sound, avoiding any injuries, with the use of protective skills, like the cross-arm technique.
- *Independence*. Patient will not be dependent on others for travel.
- *Privacy*. Helpful in accomplishment of tasks needing privacy, like banking.
- *Gracefulness*. Postural, facial, gesture training, and mannerism training lead to graceful outlook of the patient.
- *Time-saving*. Orientation to time, place, and person leads to time-saving of the patient.

Principles of orientation and mobility training:

- Where am I? Feel of the ambience and environment around, for example, garden, school, hospital, bus stop.
- Where do I have to go? Mental map of the destination, feel of the destination environment.
- How should I reach? A mental map of places and directions, appropriate use of techniques, like yardstick or human guide.

12.6 SETTING UP A LOW-VISION CLINIC

The low-vision clinic consists of anterior-posterior segment instruments, refraction kit, logMAR vision charts, contrast sensitivity charts, colour testing, field testing, and the trial sets of the devices.

The author recommends that integration of community is important for those who are having vision loss, by establishing basic low-vision clinics at the community level too. The essentials of low-vision delivery or having trained human resources and support system for a right referral pattern. The community low-vision centre should be able to identify the visually impaired patients, do a basic clinical assessment, understand their needs, and prescribe some basic magnification devices along with training. The patient can be referred to tertiary centres for advanced low-vision prescriptions; however, the follow-up can be maintained at the community set-up. The complete rehabilitation of the patient includes a teamwork of clinical and non-clinical people, like rehab personal educators, social workers, and therapists. It will not be feasible to have all the equipment; however, district hospital–level low-vision units can be sufficient to cater to population needs. The patient can return to the community centre, and the optometrist can further do counselling and training of the use of these devices.

The proposed low-vision kit for the community set-up can be:

- LogMAR chart, non-illuminated
- 2×, 3×, 4× self-illuminated hand magnifiers
- 4×, 6× stand magnifiers

- 3×, 4× monocular telescope
- 2× binocular telescopes
- Spectacle magnifiers +5, +8, +10, and +16 power
- Grey-tint filter glasses for glare control, and yellow tint for contrast enhancement
- Non-optical devices, including signature guide, reading guide, writing guide, slant reading table, under-table lamp

This basic kit will be sufficient to cater to most low-vision patients.

BIBLIOGRAPHY

1. ICD—Classification of Diseases, Functioning, and Disability. International Statistical classification of diseases, injuries and causes of death, tenth revision. Atlanta, GA: National Center for Health Statistics; 1993. Available from: www.cdc.gov/nchs/icd.htm; International Updated Sept 1 2009; Accessed on 15/07/2022.
2. Arditi A, Rosenthal B. Developing an objective definition of visual impairment. In Proceedings in Vision'96: Proceedings of the international low vision conference (pp. 331–334). Madrid: Medicare; 1998.
3. The definition of blindness under NPCB. Available from: npcb.nic.in/index1.asp?linkid=55. National Program for the Control of Blindness. Available from: www.npcb.nic.in. Accessed on 16/07/2022.
4. Dandona L, Dandona R, John RK. Estimation of blindness in India from 2000 through 2020: Implications for the blindness control policy. Natl Med J India 2001;14:327–34.
5. Virgili G, Acosta R, Grover LL, Bentley SA, Giacomelli G. Reading aids for adults with low vision. The Cochrane Database Sys Rev 2013;10:CD003303.
6. American Academy of Ophthalmology Vision Rehabilitation Committee. Preferred practice pattern guidelines. Vision rehabilitation. San Francisco, CA: American Academy of Ophthalmology; 2013. Available from: www.aao.org/ppp. Accessed on 16/07/2022.
7. Rubin GS. Demonstrating the effectiveness of low-vision rehabilitation with outcomes of the Veterans Affairs Low Vision Intervention Trial II (LOVIT II). JAMA Ophthalmol DOI: 10.1001/jamaophthalmol.2016.4778.
8. Bray N, Brand A, Taylor J, Hoare Z, Dickinson C, Edwards RT. Portable electronic vision enhancement systems in comparison with optical magnifiers for near vision activities: An economic evaluation alongside a randomized crossover trial. Acta Ophthalmol 2017 Aug;95(5):e415–23.
9. Ganesh S, Sethi S, Srivastav S, et al. Impact of low vision rehabilitation on functional vision performance of children with visual impairment. Oman J Ophthalmol 2013;6:170–4.
10. Moisseiev E, Mannis MJ. Evaluation of a portable artificial vision device among patients with low vision. JAMA Ophthalmol 2016;134:748–52.
11. Mednick Z, Jaidka A, Nesdole R, Bona M. Assessing the iPad as a tool for low-vision rehabilitation. Can J Ophthalmol 2017; 52:13–9.

12. Owsley C, McGwin G, Elgin J, Wood JM. Visually impaired drivers who use bioptic telescopes: Self-assessed driving skills and agreement with on-road driving evaluation. Invest Ophthalmol Vis Sci 2014;55:330–6.

13. Bowers AR, Sheldon SS, DeCarlo DK, Peli E. Bioptic telescope use and driving patterns of drivers with age-related macular degeneration. Trans Vis Sci Technol 2016;5:5.

14. Scott IU, Smiddy WE, Schiffman J, et al. Quality of life of low-vision patients and the impact of low-vision services. Am J Ophthalmol 1999;128: 54–62.

15. Hamade N, Hodge WG, Rakibuz-Zaman M, et al. The effects of low-vision rehabilitation on reading speed and depression in age related macular degeneration: A meta-analysis. PLoS One 2016;11:e0159254.

16. Lamoureux EL, Pallant JF, Pesudovs K, et al. The effectiveness of low-vision rehabilitation on participation in daily living and quality of life. Invest Ophthalmol Vis Sci 2007;48:1476–82.

17. Kovai V, Krishnaiah S, Shamanna BR, Thomas R, Rao GN. Barriers to accessing eye care services among visually impaired populations in rural Andhra Pradesh, South India. Indian J Ophthalmol 2007;55:365–71.

18. Binns AM, Bunce C, Dickinson C, et al. How effective is low vision service provision? A systematic review. Surv Ophthalmol 2012;57:34–65.

19. Khan SA, Shamanna B, Nuthethi R. Perceived barriers to the provision of low vision services among ophthalmologists in India. Indian J Ophthalmol 2005;53:69–75.

20. Overbury O, Wittich W. Barriers to low vision rehabilitation: The Montreal Barriers Study. Invest Ophthalmol Vis Sci 2011;52:8933–8.

13

Teleophthalmology and Digital Technologies for Primary Eye Care

KOWSALYA AKKAYASAMY AND
MOHAMMED GOWTH AMANULLAH

13.1 THE RATIONALE FOR TELEOPHTHALMOLOGY AND DIGITAL TECHNOLOGIES IN VISION CENTRES

Vision centres are primary eye care centres located in remote towns (rural areas) with a population of 50,000 to 70,000. These are the areas where patients lack access to an ophthalmologist and are unable to find the time or afford the travel expenditure to seek quality medical care.

Due to the low ophthalmologist-to-population ratio (1:100,000) in India, and with most of them practicing in urban areas, it is important to have certified allied ophthalmic personnel to provide eye care to people living in rural areas. In this context, vision centres are manned by trained and skill-certified ophthalmic technicians from the service area providing the best possible comprehensive eye care in a primary setting. Although the design of the vision centres is meant to provide primary eye care, the ocular conditions that are prevalent in the community have no differences between urban and rural areas. Hence, more skills are provided to the staff by intense training to diagnose various ocular conditions and enable delivery of appropriate treatment after thorough review by an ophthalmologist. Telemedicine-supported vision centres provide the opportunity for patients to directly interact with the consultant through the use of technology using real-time patient data.[1]

Hence, with the advancements in information technology, there are greater scopes for improvement both in the quality of diagnosis and service given to the patients visiting these vision centres. This starts by addressing the gap with the help of the ophthalmologist's opinion for every patient. This is considered ideal

DOI: 10.1201/9781003291626-13

for certain conditions, like acute conjunctivitis, allergic conjunctivitis, mild iritis, dry eyes, foreign body, glass prescription, patients for post-op cataract review, etc. For patients with chronic eye conditions like ulcers, abnormality in the fundus, increased intraocular pressure, it is mandatory to get a first-hand opinion from the ophthalmologist, and thus, they are advised to visit the ophthalmology centre for the same. The upcoming developments in artificial intelligence, especially in diagnosing chronic eye conditions like diabetic retinopathy, glaucoma, and ARMD with fundus imaging, will also lower the dependency on ophthalmologists for teleconsultation in the near future. It also provides a strong economic rationale for using deep learning systems as an assistive tool for screening DR.[2] The need for teleconsultation is built around the quality and patient safety grounds instead of depending on allied ophthalmic personnel for patient care, advice, decision, and follow-up.

From the patient care perspective, to get a consultation from the ophthalmologist is a great recourse for the patient. This will increase the service uptake and greatly influences the patient's compliance with the treatment. In modern times, technology offers a great scope for this through telemedicine. Information technology has evolved over decades to reach the current level, where it is highly simplified for adoption in the local context. The initial phase evolved through experimenting with various technologies, which include store and forward, voice chat, teleconsultation with paper case records. The recent one is electronic medical records (EMR) accommodating slit lamp photographs, fundus photographs, record of all previous visits and opinions, capturing vital signs like blood sugar levels, blood pressure, blood test indices, ocular indices like B scan, intraocular pressure, colour vision, central field tests. That the real-time video teleconsultation with the ophthalmologist who has access to the EMR of the concerned patients correctly analyzes this information for diagnosis demonstrates a great hope for connecting rural patients for eye care.

13.2 WORKFLOW AT VC AND BASE HOSPITAL

When a patient visits a vision centre, he/she gets a comprehensive ophthalmic examination done by the technician. This includes the history of presenting illness, systemic history, history of glass usage, visual acuity, IOP, refraction, muscle balance and accommodation, BP, blood sugar, anterior segment findings, fundus (undilated/dilated) findings, and diagnosis. All findings are entered into the EMR. The patient then gets a real-time video consultation with an ophthalmologist at the base hospital. For each consultation, it takes 2.5 to 3 min for the ophthalmologist to access and look into the patient's record and talk to the patient at the vision centre end. The vision centre technician orients the patient that he/she is going to interact with an ophthalmologist at the base hospital. The ophthalmologists will introduce themselves, call the patient by his/her name to reassess his/her identity, and then EMR is opened on their screen. Listening to the complaints of the patient (as presented by both the patient and the technician) and going through the EMR, the ophthalmologist advises the patient and guides the vision technician

Table 13.1 Infrastructure and Requirements to Set Up Teleophthalmology

Requirements	Base Hospital	Vision Centre
Space	4×5 ft cubicle with soundproof glass to resist noise during teleconsultation	Part of the examination room (10×12 ft)
Furniture	Table for computers, mic, speaker, and modem	Table for computers, mic, speaker, and modem
Internet connectivity	10 to 15 Mbps speed	Minimum 5 Mbps speed
Teleconsultation application	Google Hangouts, Skype, Zoom	
EMR software	Medical records are mandatory at VCs to document the finding and diagnosis of a patient and for future continuation of care. This can be both on paper and electronic. While there is a documentation and preservation issue of paper records, electronic records facilitate good documentation of the patient diagnosis and treatment recommendations more objectively. With technology becoming accessible and affordable, this is possible in all locations in the near future. This will be done with the documentation of the patients' ID and diagnosis from the drop-down menu. The data can be retrieved at any time. As the integration among primary, secondary, and tertiary hospitals happens, the record of the patient can also be retrieved anywhere from the same network. This electronic record at the vision centre level is called the vision centre management system (e.g. Aravind, LVPEI, Pellucid, and others), providing end-to-end solutions from patient registration, documentation of findings, imaging, receiving teleconsultation and e-prescriptions from the ophthalmologist, and generating reports.	
Power backup	1.5 KV invertors to ensure uninterrupted power supply	Should be part of hospital UPS

to provide more details. Prescription sent by the ophthalmologist for glasses/medicines is printed at the vision centre and handed over to the patient. The ophthalmologist also advises the patient for the precautions to be taken and next follow-up visit. This design of closing the loop from diagnosis to intervention has resulted in patient satisfaction and has benefitted a lot of patients who were unable to access primary eye care. On average, a dedicated ophthalmologist can potentially do 120–150 consultations per day. In terms of internet connectivity, 4 to 5 Mbps broadband is sufficient for the teleconsultation at one vision centre. There is always a chance for disruption in terms of connectivity, electronic device crashes, slower EMR accessibility at either ends, but most of the time, it works smoothly.

13.2.1 Training

To make the technology work and provide the desired results, it is important to educate about the purpose and importance of teleconsultation and also develop competent skills among vision centre technicians, ophthalmologists, and support staff to use it. Formal training needs to be arranged to develop a detailed understanding about:

- Handling computers and checking the mic, web camera, and internet connectivity installed at vision centres.
- The vision centre electronic medical record software installed at vision centres.
- Entering the patient details (name, age, residence, MRN, UIN) for registration, examination findings, and uploading the fundus images in the electronic medical record (EMR) software.
- Enabling hassle-free teleconsultation between the ophthalmologist and the patients.
- Generating reports—on the outpatients, refraction done, glass prescription, identification of other ocular pathologies, spectacles sale, and daily cash collection reports.
- The barriers in information technology, the disruptions in connectivity, and how to escalate it to the base hospital professional support team.

13.3 ROLES AND RESPONSIBILITIES

Vision Technician
- Orient and brief every new patient about the teleconsultation process. Consent should be obtained from every patient for the process.
- Document the history (presenting eye complaints, systemic) and ocular examination findings in the EMR.
- Facilitate hassle-free teleconsultation between the ophthalmologist and the patients.
- Answer the queries raised by the ophthalmologist to perform an additional examination on demand by the ophthalmologist (e.g. repeat IOP, fundus imaging, dilate RR, colour vision, etc.)

Teleconsultant Ophthalmologist
- Available during the committed time period for teleconsultation.
- Introduce themselves as the ophthalmologist with their name and the location from where they are interacting with the patients.

Workflow at the Vision Centre:

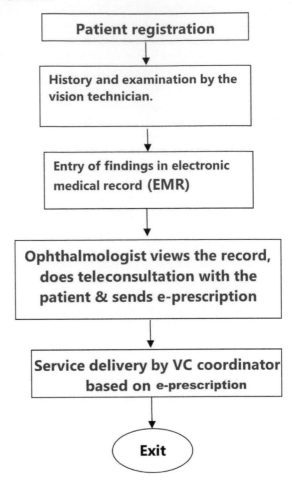

Figure 13.1 Workflow at the vision centre.

- Interact with the patient clearly in the local language after going through the findings documented in the EMR.
- Ensuring that the correct EMR coding is done for every registered patient.
- Providing E-prescription and advice based on the EMR and teleconsultation with the patient.
- In case of need of further interventions, communicate the need for visiting the base hospital.
- Build trust in the vision centre model through their conversation with the patients.
- Motivate the vision technicians for acquiring better diagnostic skills; if need be, teach them and correct them.

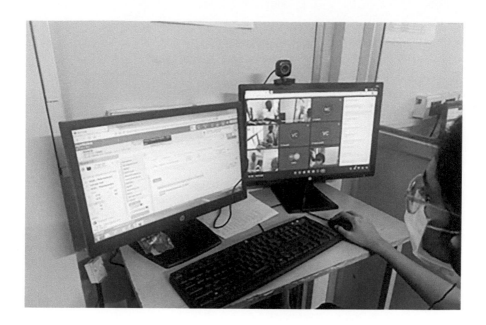

Photo 13.1 Teleophthalmology unit at Aravind Eye Hospital, Madurai. Digital image, accessed 5 October 2022.

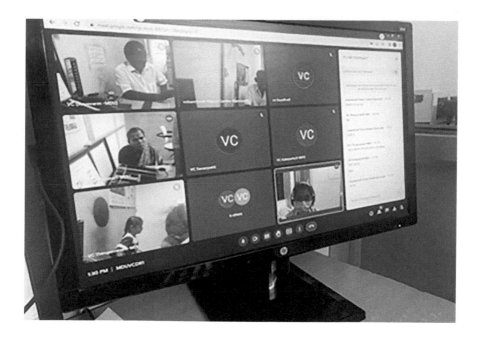

Photo 13.2 Videoconferencing for teleophthalmology via Google Meet. Digital image accessed 5 October 2022.

IT Personnel
- Setting up the hardware, software, and printers.
- Ensuring continuous internet connectivity.
- Training the doctors and vision technicians for using electronic medical records, teleconsultation process, and solving minor issues.
- Solving operational issues related to hardware, software, and connectivity.
- Customizing the reports as and when required.

13.3.1 Building Awareness in the Community

Although creating awareness about eye care happens in the community through various approaches, it is important to convey to the community that teleconsultation helps the people in accessing an ophthalmologist from their village. This can be done through various awareness programs in schools, women's development programs, panchayat meetings, etc. This will help in increasing awareness about vision centres among the service area population. Sharing the model/process through the video of how the teleconsultation happens at vision centres can build trust among the community for this process of consultation.

13.4 BENEFITS OF TELEOPHTHALMOLOGY AND DIGITAL TECHNOLOGIES

With the established teleophthalmology and continuous consultation between vision centres and base hospital, there will be increased trust among the patients for this system as ophthalmologists directly interact with them.

- It is the base hospital ophthalmologist's responsibility to prescribe medicines, advise spectacles, recommend surgery, or refer the patient to the base hospital for further investigation.
- Treatment of the ocular emergencies and anterior segment pathologies[3] is possible with telemedicine, as otherwise, the patient may choose a nearby traditional healer over visiting the ophthalmologist at the hospital, which consumes time and money.
- Irrational usage of certain eye drops which could be harmful for the patients can be prevented, and the patient can be counselled to visit only certified ophthalmologists for treatment.
- Further worsening or progression of multiple eye pathologies is prevented at the right time by appropriate intervention. This will otherwise be ignored or mistreated.
- Loss to follow-up can be prevented for patients, as they can visit these vision centres instead of every time coming to the base hospital. Regression/progression of the condition can be screened and treatment stopped/changed/dosage increased/dosage decreased accordingly.
- As and when a patient is consulted, there is a scope for improvement in the diagnosing quality of a vision technician, as the teleconsultant ophthalmologists ask for clarifications.

- Thus, teleconsultation serves as continuous education for the staff and also helps in monitoring the quality of work.
- The scope of diagnosing chronic eye conditions like diabetic retinopathy, glaucoma, and other posterior segment ocular pathologies increases with sharing of fundus images through EMR and getting opinions from teleconsultant ophthalmologists.
- Nearly 15% of the patients are referred to the base hospital, and thus, this reduces base hospital visits significantly. It increases trust and satisfaction[4] among the patients and significantly reduces the cost and carbon footprint[5] for patients visiting the base hospital.
- This helps in achieving both closing the service loop and monitoring the standalone vision centres.
- Referrals can be electronically tracked through a unique patient identification number, and the non-compliant patients can be followed up for treatment.
- Telemedicine linked with EMR ensures the availability of detailed case records for future reference to provide continuous tracking and treatment for the patients. The availability and accessibility to older records on EMR help diagnose and treat chronic/recurrent conditions.
- IT also helps in monitoring day-to-day operations, like attendance of the staff, patient attendance in real time, ordering of glasses online, and supply chain management of vision centres.
- During the pandemic situation, it helps us track our staff and ensure that they are safe, by having continuous interactions. The staff can be updated on the safety measures, and it can be ensured if they are compliant with them.[6]
- Online continuing medical education (CME) programs can be organized to refresh their knowledge post-lockdown. Recent updates in the diagnosis and treatment guidelines can be appropriately communicated and taught by certified ophthalmologists to the staff.

Benefits to the Resident Ophthalmologists at the Base Hospital

1. Daily quality consultation with a large volume of patients and correlating the findings for arriving at a diagnosis in a short period of time helps in improving the diagnostic skills of the ophthalmologist.
2. It adds to the knowledge about common ophthalmic conditions and their treatment guidelines. It indirectly ensures that the ophthalmologists at the base hospital are updated and aware about the latest guidelines practiced.
3. It enables ophthalmologists to follow up the patients aptly, thereby helping them understand the epidemiology of the disease course of the illness, duration of illness, and rate of recovery as per the latest treatment guidelines followed.
4. The ophthalmologist at the base hospital can ensure that the treatment administered to the patient at the vision centre is appropriate by analyzing the response to the treatment through a quick review check-up as advised on the patient's first visit. Since vision centres are nearby the patient's residence, there will be a decreased dropouts and loss to follow-ups than the usual numbers when the patients would have to travel longer distances.

5. Any addition or changes to the previous treatment can be made at the correct time. This adds to the treating ophthalmologist's efficiency.
6. It helps the ophthalmologists to be part of screening the causes for preventable blindness, like cataract, glaucoma, diabetic retinopathy (fundus photograph), at remote and rural areas.

13.4.1 Financial Sustainability

As a rural patient gets an opportunity to talk to a doctor, ensuring teleconsultation for all the patients visiting vision centre builds trust in the community. Backup by an ophthalmologist with teleconsultation ensures the quality of eye care to the rural population. This results in more patients turning to the OPD and increased uptake of services, like acceptance of glasses, cataract surgeries, and specialty treatment at the base hospital. The cost of travel, attender visits, food, and loss of wages will be saved and spent in the community.

Quality
- Quality of diagnosis is checked by the ophthalmologists in the base hospital through clinical auditing.
- Quality in videoconferencing and audio is maintained by a dedicated IT team daily.
- The quality of fundus photo images is usually checked by the consultant in the base hospital and clinical in charge on a weekly basis.

13.5 CONCLUSION

Approximately 25% of the population needs eye care, and at least 80% can be addressed at the primary level through vision centres or similar approaches. These centres, by design, are manned by the ophthalmic assistants or mid-level ophthalmic personnel. Using telemedicine and electronic records, patients can get opinions from an ophthalmologist. This helps them in receiving the correct advice on time and increased acceptance. It also reduces travel costs for rural patients. Especially during pandemic times, telemedicine provides great support in accessing eye care and cutting down costs. Similar to any other field, adopting communication technology to rural eye care increases the scope for universal coverage. From the National Medical Commission, a "Guidelines for Practice of Telemedicine in India" has been introduced recently and will be very helpful for those who want to relocate and practice telemedicine in their locations.

ACKNOWLEDGEMENT

Dr T. Kumaragurupari, PhD, Chief Librarian, Aravind Eye Hospital, Madurai
   Dr Shreya Jain, Resident, Aravind Eye Hospital, Madurai

REFERENCES

1. Komal S, Radhakrishnan N, Vardhan SA, Prajna NV. Effectiveness of a tele-ophthalmology vision centre in treating corneal disorders and its associated economic benefits. Cornea 2022;41:688–91.
2. Xie Y, Nguyen QD, Hamzah H, Lim G, Bellemo V, Gunasekeran DV, et al. Artificial intelligence for teleophthalmology-based diabetic retinopathy screening in a national programme: an economic analysis modelling study. Lancet Digit Health 2020;2:e240–e249.
3. Misra N, Khanna RC, Mettla AL, Marmamula S, Rathi VM, Das AV. Role of teleophthalmology to manage anterior segment conditions in vision centres of south India: EyeSmart study-I. Indian J Ophthalmol 2020;68:362–67.
4. Host BK, Turner AW, Muir J. Real-time teleophthalmology video consultation: an analysis of patient satisfaction in rural Western Australia. Clin Exp Optom 2018;101:129–34.
5. Venkatesh R, van Landingham SW, Khodifad AM, Haripriya A, Thiel CL, Ramulu P, et al. Carbon footprint and cost-effectiveness of cataract surgery. Curr Opin Ophthalmol 2016;27:82–8.
6. Muralikrishnan J, Christy JS, Srinivasan K, Subburaman GB, Shukla AG, Venkatesh R, et al. Access to eye care during the COVID-19 pandemic, India. Bull World Health Organ 2022;100:135–43.
7. Khanna RC, Sabherwal S, Sil A, Gowth M, Dole K, Kuyyadiyil S, et al. Primary eye care in India—the vision centre model. Indian J Ophthalmol 2020;68:333–39.

Index

Note: Page numbers in *italics* indicate a figure and page numbers in **bold** indicate a table on the corresponding page.

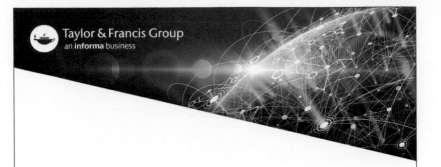